Deep Learning Identifies Brain Tumor Subregions in MR Images

By

B. Srinivas

ABSTRACT

The most precious human life is threatened by a very fatal disease that is brain tumor and it is a challenging task on the part of a doctor to diagnose the brain tumor precisely and timely. An abnormal growth of cells in the brain causes tumor and is mostly diagnosed using Magnetic Resonance Imaging (MRI). The MRI is widely used to diagnose various tissue abnormalities, detecting tumors, and evaluating residual as well as recurrent tumors. The manual and traditional medical image analysis procedures are very laborious, time-consuming, involved with slice-by-slice procedures, and the results are dependent on the experience of the radiologist and their subjective decision making. Even though there are recent developments in semi-automatic and fully-automatic image processing algorithms for removing noise from MR images, classification and segmentation of brain tumor in MR image, there are still numerous challenges mainly due to the high variation of MRI brain tumor structure in size, shape, regularity, location and their heterogeneous appearance. In addition, the tumor regions comprise discontinuities due to aggressive tumor infiltration making the medical image analysis more complex, hence resulting in poor diagnosis. Recently, due to the best performance of Deep Learning (DL) methods, specifically Convolutional Neural Networks (CNNs), in several challenges of biomedical image analysis, their popularity among researchers has increased. In traditional methods, hand crafted features are extracted whereas representative complex features are learnt directly by the CNNs automatically from the data itself. In this thesis, CNN based methods are used for the denoising, classification and segmentation of brain tumor MR images. The Thesis begins with the investigation of efficient deep learning model that avoids the iterative optimization procedure to improve both performance and computational efficiency for denoising of brain tumor images.

The prior knowledge of image based methods for denoising have the major drawbacks: i) these methods generally involve a complex optimization problem in the testing stage to make the denoising process time-consuming and high performance is hardly achieved without sacrificing computational efficiency, ii) the models are nonconvex and involve several manually chosen parameters, providing some leeway to boost denoising performance. A discriminative learning method, that is, deep

i

learning model (DnCNN) is implemented to get rid of the iterative optimization procedure in the test phase. A DeepCNN model is proposed and its performance is compared to traditional filters and pretrained DnCNN in terms of PSNR in dB, SSIM, MSE, and MAE. The proposed DeepCNN method is shown to be the best method for reducing noise when image gets corrupted by either Gaussian or speckle noise with known and unknown noise levels.

The second contribution of the research work is the development of an MRI brain tumor classification model based on Transfer Learning (TL) and hybrid methods for better classification of the brainr tumor. The proposed TL model with ADAM optimizer has shown better performance accuracy and error rate (97.91 % & 2.08 %) than that of SGDM optimizer (96.25 % & 3.75 %). Also, several hybrid models by combining CNN-features with machine learning classifiers like KNN, CNN, SVM, Discriminant analysis, Naive Bayes, Ensemble, and Tree are considered for classification and their performance is evaluated based on metrics like accuracy, F1 score, and error rate. Among all hybrid models, the proposed CNN-KNN model has provided the highest classification accuracy of 96.25 %.

The third and major contribution of this research work is the development of reliable deep learning models for automatic segmentation and accurate extraction of brain tumor subregions. Due to complexity of medical images, applying single modality of the image and using single DL model are not enough to extract the brain tumor subregions. Because generally tumor core is inside of whole tumor, and enhancing tumor is part of tumor core, reliable deep learning models have been proposed for automatic segmentation. The models are constructed based on U-net and VGG16 models architectures. Instead of using all MRI modalities, T2 and FLAIR image data is used for whole tumor segmentation using 23 layers DL model. Only T1c image data is used for tumor core and enhancing tumor segmentation using 18 layers DL model to accelerate training. The whole tumor is segmented primarily from T2 images and FLAIR is used to cross-check the extension of the edema and discriminate it against ventricles and other fluid-filled structures. Tumor core and enhancing tumor are both segmented by evaluating hyper-intensities in T1c images. The proposed models have produced outperforming results in terms of dice similarity index, Jaccard similarity index, accuracy, sensitivity, and specificity. The experimental results on testing dataset of BraTS 2018 database, the proposed DL models automatically detected the brain tumor nearly with 99.62 % accuracy on an average in comparison with k-means and fuzzy c-means models. And also the proposed model and methodology have achieved outperforming results with average dice coefficients of 0.9670, 0.9281, 0.9152 and Jaccard coefficients of 0.9374, 0.8835, 0.8471 for Tumor Core (TC), Enhancing Tumor (ET), and Whole Tumor (WT) respectively.

From the experimental results, it is concluded that the brain tumor subregions ET, TC, and WT are extracted and located precisely. In the clinical practice, this pathology system assists the radiologist to detect size, location, and shape of the brain tumor accurately and hence the radiologist or a doctor can take consistent decisions, plan the best possible treatment so that the patient survival rate is improved.

CONTENTS

Page No

Abstract   i

List of Figures   viii

List of Tables   xv

List of Abbreviations   xvii

List of Symbols   xxi

Chapter 1   Introduction   1

1.1 Introduction   1

1.2 Aim and Objectives of the thesis   4

1.3 Literature survey   5

     1.3.1 Research gaps   5

1.4 Technical Approach   17

1.5 Applications of the thesis   20

1.6 Organization of the thesis   21

Chapter 2   Introduction to brain tumor and database   22

2.1 Introduction   22

2.2 Brain tumors   22

     2.2.1 Types of brain tumors   24

         2.2.1.1 Cell type   24

         2.2.1.2 Grades of Tumor   24

     2.2.2 Causes of brain tumors   25

     2.2.3 Symptoms of brain tumors   25

     2.2.4 Statistics on brain tumors   26

2.3 Medical brain imaging   26

     2.3.1 Tumor subregions   28

2.4 BraTS database   29

     2.4.1 Clinical relevance   29

     2.4.2 Segmentation of gliomas in pre-operative MRI scans   30

     2.4.3 Imaging data description   31

     2.4.4 Comparison with previous BraTS database   32

     2.4.5 Previous BraTS challenges   32

     2.4.6 Data organizing committee and contributors   32

2.5 Conclusions   33

Chapter 3   Denoising of Brain Tumor MR Image   34

3.1 Introduction   34

3.2 Noise   34

    3.2.1 Significance of noise   35

    3.2.2 Different types of noise in medical images   35

       3.2.2.1 Gaussian noise   36

       3.2.2.2 Salt and pepper noise   36

       3.2.2.3 Speckle noise   36

       3.2.2.4 Poisson noise   37

3.3 Image denoising using traditional filters   38

3.4 Brain tumor MR image denoising using DnCNN   40

    3.4.1 Architecture of pretrained DnCNN model   40

    3.4.2 Image denoising using DnCNN   41

3.5 Brain tumor MR image denoising using proposed DeepCNN model   43

    3.5.1 Architecture of proposed deep learning model (DeepCNN)   43

    3.5.2 Image denoising using proposed DeepCNN   43

3.6 Performance evaluation metrics   45

3.7 Experimental results and discussions   47

3.8 Conclusions   69

Chapter 4   Brain Tumor MR Image Classification using Transfer Learning   70

4.1 Introduction   70

4.2 Introduction to Artificial Neural Network (ANN)   71

    4.2.1 Basics of Artificial Neural Networks   71

    4.2.2 Multilayer networks   73

4.3 Convolutional Neural Networks (CNN)   74

    4.3.1 Layers of CNNs   75

       4.3.1.1 Image Input Layer   75

       4.3.1.2 Convolutional Layer   76

       4.3.1.3 Batch Normalization Layer   79

       4.3.1.4 ReLU Layer   79

4.3.1.5 Pooling Layers   80

4.3.1.6 Dropout Layer   80

4.3.1.7 Fully Connected Layer   80

4.3.1.8 Output Layers   81

4.3.2 Activation Functions   82

4.4 Optimization with back propagation in neural networks   85

4.4.1 Optimizers   86

4.4.1.1 Stochastic gradient descent   86

4.4.1.2 Stochastic gradient descent with momentum   87

4.4.1.3 Root Mean Square Propagation (RMSProp)   88

4.4.1.4 Adaptive moment estimation (Adam)   88

4.4.2 Back propagation   89

4.4.3 Loss functions   90

4.3.3.1 Mean Square Error (MSE) loss function   91

4.3.3.2 Cross entropy loss function   91

4.3.3.3 Weighted cross entropy   92

4.3.3.4 Dice similarity coefficient loss function   92

4.5 Transfer Learning (TL)   92

4.5.1 Architecture of Alexnet   94

4.5.2 TL method and methodology   95

4.5.3 TL features with ML classifier (Hybrid models)   98

4.6 Performance evaluation metrics   100

4.7 Experimental results and discussion   100

4.7.1 Brain tumor classification with TL model   100

4.7.2 Brain tumor classification with hybrid models   104

4.7.3 Comparison of TL model with hybrid models   108

4.8 Conclusions   111

**Chapter 5 Sub regions Segmentation of brain tumor of MR   112
images**

5.1 Introduction   112

5.2 Existing segmentation methods   113

5.2.1 Thresholding methods   113

5.2.2 Region based segmentation   114

5.2.3 Edge detection   114

5.2.4 Watershed segmentation   115

5.2.5 Clustering based algorithm   116

5.2.6 Artificial Neural Network   117

5.3 Algorithms for brain tumor MR image segmentation   118

5.3.1 k-means algorithm   118

5.3.2 Fuzzy c-means clustering algorithm   119

5.3.3 Proposed deep learning models   120

5.3.3.1 Algorithmic description of brain tumor MR image subregions segmentation   121

5.3.3.2 Methodology of brain tumor MR image subregions segmentation   122

5.3.3.3 Deep Learning model architecture   123

5.4 Performance evaluation metrics   128

5.5 Experimental results and discussions   130

5.5.1 Brain tumor MR image segmentation using k-means clustering algorithm   130

5.5.2 Brain tumor MR image segmentation using fuzzy c-means clustering   133

5.5.3 MRI brain tumor segmentation using proposed deep learning models   136

5.6 Segmentation of brain tumor subregions in MR image using DL models   147

5.7 Conclusions   158

Chapter 6   Conclusions and future scope of the work   160

References   162

List of Publications relevant to the Ph.D. work   180

LIST OF FIGURES

Page No

Fig. 2.1   Brain tumor of MR images. a) LGG (benign) image b) HGG   23
           (malignant) image.

Fig. 2.2   Various orientations of MRI sequence modalities. a) Axial   27
           b) Sagittal c) Coronal.

Fig. 2.3   MRI sequence modalities. a) Fluid Attenuated Inversion   27
           Recovery (FLAIR) image b) T1-weighted image c) T1-
           Contrast enhancement (T1c) image d) T2-weighted image.

Fig. 2.4   Subregions of HGG (malignant) brain tumor of MR image.   28
           FLAIR image (left),   Ground truth image (right).

Fig. 2.5   Sub-regions of LGG (benign) brain tumor of MR image.   29
           FLAIR image (left), Ground truth image (right).

Fig. 2.6   Tumor structures present on the image patches interpreted in 31
           different modalities (top left) and the final labels for the
           whole dataset (right). Image patches shown (left to right): the
           WT visible in FLAIR (A), the tumor core visible in T2 (B),
           the enhancing tumor structures visible in T1c (blue),
           surrounding the cystic/necrotic components of the core
           (green) (C). Final labels of the tumor structures generated
           after combining the segmentations (D): edema (yellow), non-
           enhancing solid core (red), necrotic/cystic core (green),
           enhancing core (blue).

Fig. 3.1   Block diagram of image denoising with various traditional   38
           filters.

Fig. 3.2   Architecture of DnCNN model.   41

Fig. 3.3   Framework of image denoising with pretrained convolutional   42
           neural networks (DnCNNs).

Fig. 3.4   Framework of image denoising with proposed DeepCNN.   45

Fig. 3.5   Brain tumor MR image denoising with various Gaussian   50
           noise level range from 5 to 50 (from Sl.No. 1 to 10).
           a) Original images b) Noisy images c) Pretrained DnCNN
           denoised images d) Proposed DeepCNN denoised images
           e) Gaussian filter denoised images f) Bilateral filter denoised
           images g) Adaptive filter denoised images h) Guided filter
           denoised images.

Fig. 3.6   Plot of PSNR values versus Gaussian noise level for various   53
           denoising methods.

Fig. 3.7   Plot of SSIM values versus Gaussian noise level for various   53
            denoising methods.

Fig. 3.8   Plot of MSE values versus Gaussian noise level for various   54
            denoising methods.

Fig. 3.9   Plot of MAE values versus Gaussian noise level for various   55
            denoising methods.

Fig. 3.10   Denoising of Brain tumor MR image corrupted with various   58
            speckle noise level range from 5 to 50 (from Sl.No. 1 to 10).
            a) Original images b) Noisy images c) Denoised images
            using Pretrained DnCNN   d) Proposed DeepCNN denoised
            images e) Gaussian filter denoised images f) Bilateral filter
            denoised images g) Adaptive filter denoised images
            h) Guided filter denoised images.

Fig. 3.11   Plot of PSNR values versus speckle noise level for various   61
            denoising methods.

Fig. 3.12   Plot of SSIM values versus speckle noise level for various   61
            denoising methods.

Fig. 3.13   Plot of MSE values versus speckle noise level for various   62
            denoising methods

Fig. 3.14   Plot of MAE values versus speckle noise level for various   62
            denoising methods.

Fig. 3.15   Brain tumor MR image denoising with Gaussian noise of   63
            level 15. a) Original image b) Noisy image c) Pretrained
            DnCNN denoised images d) Proposed DeepCNN denoised
            images e) Gaussian filter denoised images f) Bilateral filter
            denoised images g) Adaptive filter denoised images
            h) Guided filter denoised images.

Fig. 3.16   Brain tumor MR image denoising with salt and pepper noise   64
            level 15. a) Original image b) Noisy image c) Pretrained
            DnCNN denoised images d) Proposed DeepCNN denoised
            images e) Gaussian filter denoised images f) Bilateral filter
            denoised images g) Adaptive filter denoised images
            h) Gduided filter denoised images.

Fig. 3.17   Brain tumor MR image denoising with Poisson noise level of   65
             15. a) Original image b) Noisy image c) Pretrained DnCNN
             denoised images d) Proposed DeepCNN denoised images
             e) Gaussian filter denoised images f) Bilateral filter denoised
             images g) Adaptive filter denoised images h) Guided filter
             denoised images.

Fig. 3.18   Brain tumor MR image denoising with speckle noise level of   66
             15. a) Original image b) Noisy image c) Pretrained DnCNN
             denoised images d) Proposed DeepCNN denoised images
             e) Gaussian filter denoised images f) Bilateral filter denoised
             images g) Adaptive filter denoised images h) Guided filter
             denoised images.

Fig. 3.19   PSNR performance comparison of various denoising methods.   67

Fig. 3.20   SSIM performance comparison of various denoising methods.   67

Fig. 3.21   PSNR (dB) performance comparison of proposed DeepCNN   68
             for Gaussian and speckle noise.

Fig. 3.22   PSNR (dB) performance comparison of proposed DeepCNN   68
             for Gaussian and speckle noise.

Fig. 3.23   SSIM performance comparison of proposed DeepCNN for   69
             Gaussian and speckle noise.

Fig. 4.1   Biological neuron.   72

Fig. 4.2   Artificial neuron.   72

Fig. 4.3   Feedforward neural network having one hidden layer.   73

Fig. 4.4   Single layer network   74

Fig. 4.5   Convolutional operation.   76

Fig. 4.6   Dilated convolutional operation.   77

Fig. 4.7   Zero padding operation.   78

Fig. 4.8   Sigmoid function.   83

Fig. 4.9   Tanh function.   83

Fig. 4.10   ReLU function.   84

Fig. 4.11   Leaky ReLU function   84

Fig. 4.12   Left is gradient descent without momentum, right is the   87
             gradient descent with momentum.

Fig. 4.13   Backpropagation of   for   .   90

Fig. 4.14   AlexNet   94

Fig. 4.15   Framework of transfer learning model (Fine tuning of Alexnet   95
model).

Fig. 4.16   Architecture of modified Alexnet (Transfer learning).   96

Fig. 4.17   An interactive visualization of alexnet architecture.   97

Fig. 4.18   Modified last three layers of transfer learning model.   97

Fig. 4.19   Block diagram of proposed hybrid model.   98

Fig. 4.20   Frame work of CNN-KNN image classification.   99

Fig. 4.21   Training images of 16 random images from training dataset.   101

Fig. 4.22   Training process of transfer learning model.   101

Fig. 4.23   Testing images of 16 random images from testing dataset.   102

Fig. 4.24   Testing images of 16 random images with prediction   103
percentage from testing dataset.

Fig. 4.25   Confusion matrices of proposed TL model a) with SGDM   103
optimizer b) with ADAM optimizer.

Fig. 4.26   Training options of CNN-KNN model.   105

Fig. 4.27   Weights of first convolutional layer.   106

Fig. 4.28   Features of the first convolutional layer.   106

Fig. 4.29   Features of the second convolutional layer.   107

Fig. 4.30   Features of the fully connected (dense) layer.   107

Fig. 4.31   Plot of false negative versus various classification models.   108

Fig. 4.32   Plot of accuracy versus various classification models.   109

Fig. 4.33   Plot of error rate versus various classification models.   110

Fig. 4.34   Plot between F1 score and various classification models.   110

Fig. 4.35   Plot of sensitivity versus various classification models.   111

Fig. 5.1   Segmentation of Glioma subregions using proposed   123
methodology.

Fig. 5.2   Architecture of proposed deep learning model with auto-   124
            encoder structure.

Fig. 5.3   Architecture of proposed 23 layers DL model for Whole   126
            Tumor segmentation.

Fig. 5.4   Architecture of proposed 18 layers DL model for Tumor Core   127
            and Enhancing Tumor segmentation.

Fig. 5.5   Brain tumor MRI segmentation using k-means clustering.   132
            a) Original images (FLAIR) b) Clustered image 1 c) Clustered
            image 2 d) Segmented images e) Ground truth images.

Fig. 5.6   Brain tumor MR image segmentation using fuzzy c-means   135
            clustering algorithm. a) Original images (FLAIR) b) Clustered
            image 1 c) Clustered image 2 d) Segmented images e) Ground
            truth images.

Fig. 5.7   False Negatives (FN) of a patient Brats18_TCIA08_167_1   138
            using proposed DL model.

Fig. 5.8   False Negatives (FN) of k-means, fuzzy c-means clustering   139
            and proposed DL model.

Fig. 5.9   Segmented images of 10 MRI brain tumor patients using   139
            proposed DL model.

Fig. 5.10   Segmentation results comparison of k-means, fuzzy c-means   140
            Clustering and Deep Learning models. a) Original Image
            b) Ground truth image c) K-means segmented image d) Fuzzy
            C-means segmented image e) Deep Learning Model
            segmented image.

Fig. 5.11   Accuracy comparison of k-means, fuzzy c-means and   143
            proposed DL model for 10 images.

Fig. 5.12   Error rate comparison of k-means, fuzzy c-means and   144
            proposed DL model for 10 images.

Fig. 5.13   Dice similarity coefficients comparison of K means, fuzzy c-   144
            means and proposed DL model for 10 images.

Fig. 5.14   Jaccard similarity coefficients comparison of K means, fuzzy   145
            c-means and proposed DL model for 10 images.

Fig. 5.15   Average accuracy of k-means, fuzzy c-means and proposed   145
            DL model.

Fig. 5.16   Average error rate of k-means, fuzzy c-means and proposed   146
            DL model.

Fig. 5.17   Average dice similarity coefficients of k-means, fuzzy c-means   146
             and proposed DL model.

Fig. 5.18   Average Jaccard similarity coefficients of k-means, fuzzy   147
             c-means and proposed DL model.

Fig. 5.19   Brain Tumor segmentation of patient name Brats18_2013_3_1   149
             using proposed deep learning models. Images show in first row
             a to d: T1-weighted image, T2-weighted FLAIR image, T1-
             Constrast image; from second row e to h: Ground truths of
             whole tumor (WT), tumor core (TC), enhancing tumor (ET),
             all sub-regions combination (All); from third row i to l:
             Prediction of whole tumor (WT), tumor core (TC), enhancing
             tumor (ET), all subregions combination (All).

Fig. 5.20   Brain Tumor segmentation of patient name Brats18_2013_5_1   150
             using proposed deep learning models. Images show in first row
             a to d: T1-weighted image, T2-weighted FLAIR image, T1-
             Constrast image; from second row e to h: Ground truths of
             whole tumor (WT), tumor core (TC), enhancing tumor (ET),
             all sub-regions combination (All); from third row i to l:
             Prediction of whole tumor (WT), tumor core (TC), enhancing
             tumor (ET), all subregions combination (All).

Fig. 5.21   Brain   Tumor   segmentation   of   patient   name   151
             Brats18_CBICA_AQU_1 using proposed deep learning
             models. Images show in first row a to d: T1-weighted image,
             T2-weighted FLAIR image, T1-Constrast image; from second
             row e to h: Ground truths of whole tumor (WT), tumor core
             (TC), enhancing tumor (ET), all sub-regions combination
             (All); from third row i to l: Prediction of whole tumor (WT),
             tumor core (TC), enhancing tumor (ET), all subregions
             combination (All).

Fig. 5.22   Brain   Tumor   segmentation   of   patient   name   152
             Brats18_CBICA_BHK_1 using proposed deep learning
             models. Images show in first row a to d: T1-weighted image,
             T2-weighted FLAIR image, T1-Constrast image; from second
             row e to h: Ground truths of whole tumor (WT), tumor core
             (TC), enhancing tumor (ET), all sub-regions combination
             (All); from third row i to l: Prediction of whole tumor (WT),
             tumor core (TC), enhancing tumor (ET), all subregions
             combination (All).

Fig. 5.23   Brain   Tumor   segmentation   of   patient   name   153
             Brats18_TCIA01_147_1 using proposed deep learning models.
             Images show in first row a to d: T1-weighted image, T2-
             weighted FLAIR image, T1-Constrast image; from second row
             e to h: Ground truths of whole tumor (WT), tumor core (TC),
             enhancing tumor (ET), all sub-regions combination (All); from
             third row i to l: Prediction of whole tumor (WT), tumor core
             (TC), enhancing tumor (ET), all subregions combination (All).

Fig. 5.24   Plot of tumor core versus various models in terms of dice   158
             similarity coefficient.

Fig. 5.25   Plot of enhancing tumor versus various models in terms of dice   158
             similarity coefficient.

Fig. 5.26   Plot of whole tumor versus various models in terms of dice   158
             similarity coefficient.

LIST OF TABLES

Page No

Table 2.1   Modalities of MR image.   28

Table 3.1   Performance metrics of proposed DeepCNN, pretrained DnCNN, Gaussian, adaptive, bilateral, and guided filters with Gaussian noise from noise level 5 to 50.   51

Table 3.2   Performance metrics of proposed DeepCNN, pretrained DnCNN, Gaussian, adaptive, bilateral, and guided filters with speckle noise from various noise level 5 to 50.   59

Table 3.3   PSNR (dB)/SSIM of proposed DeepCNN, pretrained DnCNN,Gaussian, bilateral, adaptive, and guided filters for various noises with noise level 15.   66

Table 4.1   Confusion matrix of various classification models.   108

Table 4.2   Performance comparison of various classification methods.   109

Table 5.1   Layers details of original U-net, proposed DL models with 23 and 18 layers.   126

Table 5.2   Confusion matrix.   128

Table 5.3   Confusion matrix of k-means Clustering algorithm.   133

Table 5.4   Confusion matrix of Fuzzy C-means clustering.   136

Table 5.5   Confusion matrix of proposed DL model.   138

Table 5.6   Performance comparison of various segmentation methods in terms of accuracy and error rate.   141

Table 5.7   Specificity performance evaluation of various segmentation methods.   142

Table 5.8   Sensitivity performance evaluation of various segmentation methods.   142

Table 5.9   F1-score performance evaluation of various segmentation methods.   143

Table 5.10   Performance of various segmentation methods in terms of dice and Jaccard similarity coefficients.   143

Table 5.11   Performance evaluation metrics accuracy and error rate of tumor core.   154

Table 5.12   Performance evaluation metrics specificity, sensitivity, and F1-score of tumor core.   154

Table 5.13   Performance evaluation metrics accuracy and error rate of enhancing tumor.   155

Table 5.14   Performance evaluation metrics specificity, sensitivity, and F1-score of enhancing tumor.   155

Table 5.15   Comparison of dice similarity coefficient for ET, TC, and WT.   156

Table 5.16   Comparison of jaccard similarity coefficient for ET, TC, and WT.   156

Table 5.17   Comparison of dice similarity coefficient of deep learning models with other models.   157

ABBREVIATIONS

2D-DWT	2-Dimensional Discrete Wavelet Transform
2D	2-Dimmensional
3D	3-Dimmensional
ACC	Accuracy
AT	Active Tumor
AF	Adaptive Filter
ADAM	Adaptive moment estimation
ARMS	Alveolar
AD	Anistropic Diffusion
ANN	Artificial Neural Networks
AS	Astrocytoma
BN	Batch Normalization
BF	Bilateral Filter
BM3D	Block-matching and 3D filtering
BBB	Brain Blood Blurry
BTD	Brain Tumor Database
BRATS	Brain Tumor Segmentation
CBICA	Center for Biomedical Image Computing and Analytics
CNS	Central Nervous System
CMB	Cerebral microbleeds
CSF	Cerebrospinal fluid
cc	Cluster Centre
CT	Computed Tomography
CAD System	Computer Aided Diagnostic System
CRF	conditional random fields
CE	Contrast Enhancement
Conv	Convolutional layer
CNN	Convolutional Neural Network
CNN-DISCR	Convolutional Neural Network- Discriminant
CNN-NB	Convolutional Neural Network- Naive Bayes
CNN-TREE	Convolutional Neural Network-Decision Tree

CNN-ENSEMBLE	Convolutional Neural Network-Ensemble
CNN-KNN	Convolutional Neural Network-k-Nearest Neighbours
CNN-SVM	Convolutional Neural Network-Support Vector Machine
DFS	Dark Frame Subtraction
DeepCNN	Deep Convolutional Neural Network
DL	Deep Learning
DNN	Deep Neural Network
DSC	Dice Similarity Coefficient
DWI	Diffusion-Weighted MR Image
ED	Edema
ERMS	Embryonal
ET	Enhancing Tumor
FN	False Negatives
FPR	false positive rate
FP	False Positives
FFDNet	Fast and Flexible Denoising Convolutional Neural Network
DnCNN	Feed-forward Denoising Convolutional Neural Network
FLAIR	Fluid Attenuate Image Recovery
FLAIR	Fluid Attenuated Inversion Recovery
FC	Fully Connected
FCM	Fuzzy C-Means
FJP	Fuzzy Joint Points
Gad	Gadolinium
GAF	Gaussian Filter
GA	Genetic Algorithm
GBM	Glioblastoma Multiforme
GVF	Gradient Vector Flow
GPU	Graphical Processing Unit
GLCM	Grey Level Co-occurrence Matrix
GUF	Guided Filter
HD	Hausdorff
HGG	High Grade Gliomas
ISLES	Ischemic stroke lesion segmentation

JSC	Jaccard similarity Coefficient
LReLU	Leaky Rectified Linear Unit
LDA	Linear Discriminant Analysis
LGG	Low Grade Glioma
MRI	Magnetic Resonance Imaging
MAE	Mean Absolute Error
MSE	Mean Squared Error
MED	Medulloblastoma
MEN	Meningioma
MET	Metastatic
MCCNN	Multi-Cascaded CNN
NCI	National Cancer Institute
NIH	National Institutes of Health
NCR/NET	Necrotic and Non Enhancing Tumor core
NN	Neural Networks
PSNR	Peak Signal to Noise Ratio
PPR	Positive Predictive Rate
PPV	Positive Predictive Value
PET	Positron Emission Tomography
PCA	Principle Component Analysis
ReLU	Rectifier Linear Unit
RGB	Red Blue Green
ResNet	Residual Network
RMS	Rhabdomysarcoma
SE	Sensitivity
SPECT	Single Photon Emission Computed Tomography
SK-TPNN	Small Kernels Two Path CNN
SP	Specificity
SGDM	Stochastic gradient descent with momentum
SSIM	Structural Similarity index of Image
T1	T1-weighted
T1c	T1-weighted image post-contrast enhancement
T2	T2-weighted

TCIA	The Cancer Imaging Archive
TL	Transfer Learning
TN	True Negatives
TPR	True positive rate
TP	True Positives
TC	Tumor Core
VGG16	Visual Geometry Group 16
WT	Whole tumor
WHO	World Health Organization

SYMBOLS

$f()$	Activation function
b	Bias
q^{th}	Cluster center
v_q	Cluster centroids
$c(p,q)$	Contrast differences
$D(S,L)$	Cross entropy loss function
p^{th}	Data point
β	Decay rate
dB	Decibels
$\|X_p\text{-}v_q\|^2$	Euclidean distance
e	Exponential
$G(u,v)$	FCM objective function
m	Fuzziness index
$\varepsilon(w_i)$	Gradient of the loss function
g	Gray level
L_i	Ground truth label
h	Height of the filter
α	Initial learning rate
$R(a,b)$	Input images
u_j	Input layer
i	Iteration number
μ	Learning rate
$\varepsilon()$	Loss function
$l(p,q)$	Luminance differences
U	Matrix of fuzzy membership
μ	Mean
μ_{pq}	Membership function of data points to cluster centers
δ	Momentum parameter
	Neuron
width	Number of channels

C	Number of classes
K	Number of cluster centroids
n	Number of columns
n	Number of data points
R	Number of responses
m	Number of rows
	Pi
S	Predicted output
y_i	Prediction for response
D(a,b)	Segmented image
$y_r(x)$	Softmax function
σ	Standard deviation (Noise level)
r(p,q)	Structural variations
t_i	Target output
E	Termination criterion
d_{pq}	The Euclidean distance between p^{th} data points and q^{th} cluster centers
σ^2	Variance
w_j	Weights of the filters
w	Width of the filter

Chapter 1

Introduction

1.1 Introduction

The challenging task for doctors is to detect brain tumor cases precisely to save human lives. Generally, brain tumors are classified into benign and malignant and if these cases are treated early and properly, 90 % of them would get cured. There are various techniques available to detect a brain tumor but early and precise detection of tumors can increase patient survival period. For this purpose, a reliable Computer Aided Diagnostic (CAD) system is necessary which uses the advanced improvement technologies of data acquisition, processing, analysis and visualization for detection, segmentation of tumor accurately and classifying it correctly.

Brain tumor diagnosis is a crucial task and to plan for the treatment, medical images are generally used. These medical images are acquired using various technologies like Computed Tomography (CT), Magnetic Resonance Imaging (MRI), Positron Emission Tomography (PET), and X-ray, are widely used in the medical field. Among them, MR Imaging technique is commonly used for brain tumor segmentation task as well as a classification problem. Since the introduction of magnetic resonance imaging in 1970s, its utilization has been spreading increasingly. However, since there is no fully automatic detection system for brain tumors, MRIs are analyzed by human experts. This requires time and concentration, and chances of human errors more.

The characteristics of MRI include superior soft tissue differentiation, high spatial resolution, and contrast. They give rich information for biomedical research and disease diagnosis. It uses nonharmful ionizing radiation to patients. But the segmentation and classification of medical images is a very challenging task, because the MR brain tumor image is a 3D data where tumor shape, size, and location varies greatly from patient to patient. And also the tumor's boundaries have very fuzzy and irregular boundaries due to their infiltrative nature. In addition to these, brain tumor

1

MRI data obtained from clinical scans or synthetic databases are inherently complex. MRI devices and protocols used for acquisition can vary dramatically from scan to scan imposing intensity biases and other variations for each different slice of the image in the dataset. The need for several modalities to effectively segment tumor subregions even adds to this complexity.

Image segmentation is a critical step for the MR images to be used in brain tumor analysis. Image segmentation is to partition an image into its coherent parts. These partitions after the segmentation have similar characteristics such as color, texture etc. Some of the most widely known image segmentation methods in the literature are clustering based methods, edge based methods, threshold based methods, region based methods, and other trainable models. Although image segmentation makes an image easier to analyze, it actually does not convey high level information. In order to interpret the high level information of an image, these segmented parts should be classified. Semantic image segmentation combines segmentation with per pixel classification. In other words, in semantic segmentation, each pixel is assigned a class label and when those pixels are combined, they correspond to segments in the image. This type of approach is considered to extract the segmentation subregions of MRI brain tumor. Image segmentation can be categorized as unsupervised and supervised segmentation.

In unsupervised segmentation, the inputs are provided but ground truths are not provided by the user for training the algorithm and user interaction is needed. So, the algorithm learns by itself or it does not need any supervision. Supervised segmentation methods need input and a user interaction for the segmentation. User needs to either mark a region or it needs to provide the correct segmentation output (ground truth or mask) to the algorithm.

In order to train the deep learning algorithms, both supervised and unsupervised learning can be used. Generally segmentation is followed by classification in non-convolutional neural network methods but this thesis focuses on using Deep Learning (DL). The proposed models and methodologies used here is to increase the patient's life span by diagnosing the enhancing tumor for HGG cases at an earlier stage. This can be achieved by performing classification prior to segmentation as HGG cases have malignant tendency. Image classification is to label

2

an image or a part of an image with the corresponding classes based on its features. The classical approach for classification has two main steps. The first one is the feature extraction in which important information related to the class labels are obtained. Edges, corners and color information are only a few examples for these features. The second step is to decide which class those features belong to. This step is carried out by machine learning algorithms. Features are actually high dimensional vectors that reside in a feature space and represent the object or content. Machine learning algorithms strives to separate the feature space into meaningful regions (hyper planes) that correspond to classes. If the feature vector of an object is in one of these regions, then that object is predicted as the corresponding class. On the other hand, Convolutional Neural Network (CNN) is an example of supervised learning algorithm which requires labels of the objects during training.

Automatic segmentation of MRI brain tumor subregions has the following advantages: i) The segmented subregions of brain tumor eliminates confounding structures from other brain tumor tissues and therefore provides a more accurate segmentation for the subregions. ii) The accurate delineation is crucial in radiotherapy or surgery planning, from which not only brain tumor extent has been outlined but also surrounding healthy tissues has been excluded carefully in order to avoid injury to other parts during the therapy. iii) Segmentation of longitudinal MRI scans can efficiently monitor brain tumor recurrence, growth or shrinkage. In current clinical practice, the segmentation is still relied on manual delineation by radiologists. The manual segmentation is a very labor-intensive task, which normally involves slice-by-slice procedures, and the results are greatly dependent on radiologist's experience and their subjective decision making. Moreover, reproducible results are difficult to achieve even by the same clinical expert. For a multi-modal, multi-institutional and longitudinal clinical trial, a fully automatic, objective and reproducible segmentation method is highly in demand to assist the radiologist. To improve the diagnosis made by a radiologist further, the state of the art algorithms proposed based on deep learning concepts are used to extract subregions of an MR image.

To achieve better performance metrics by image classification and segmentation, the image must be noise free. So, image denoising is a fundamental computer vision task that yields images with reduced noise, and improves the execution of other tasks, such as image classification and image restoration. Deep

3

learning based image denoisers have performances that are equivalent to or better than those of conventional denoising techniques such as BM3D (Kostadin Dabov et al., 2007). These deep denoisers typically train their networks by minimizing the Mean Squared Error (MSE) between denoised and the original (noiseless) images. Thus, it is crucial to have high quality noiseless image for high performance deep learning denoisers. So far, deep neural network denoisers have been successful since high quality camera sensors and abundant light allow the acquisition of high quality, almost noiseless 2D images in daily environment tasks. Thus, acquiring ground truth data with newly developed MRI scanners seems challenging without compromising the patient's safety.

In recent years, several automatic or semiautomatic methods have been proposed for diagnosis and classification of brain tumors (Shin H C et al., 2016). For low-level extraction of features Grey Level Co-occurrence Matrix (GLCM) (Sebastian V et al., 2012) has been used commonly and neural networks are used (Othman M et al., 2011, Sun X et al., 2017) to handle complex texture of brain tumor. To model new complex and nonlinear relationships between the input and output layers, deep learning is introduced. This is an extension of traditional neural networks and formed by adding extra hidden layers to the network model. Deep learning has gained the researcher's interest due to its good performance and seems to be the best solution for medical image analysis applications like image denoising (Zhang K et al., 2017), segmentation, and classification (Zhang Y D et al., 2015). Presently, there are various DL architectures and Convolutional Neural Networks (CNNs) is the architecture which performs complex operations using convolutional filters.

1.2 Aim and objectives of the thesis

The aim of this research is to implement automatic image processing techniques to precisely detect, classify, and segment the brain tumor tissue subregions from multi-modal MR images. This thesis focuses on Convolutional Neural Network models and methodologies for noise removal, classification, and extraction of subregions from brain tumor MR images.

To achieve this aim, the following objectives are considered.

i) Development of a DeepCNN based denoising model for different types of known and blind image denoising applications.

ii) Development of transfer learning and hybrid models (CNN-KNN, CNN-SVM, CNN-DISCR, CNN-NB, CNN-ENSEMBLE, CNN-TREE) for classification of brain tumor MR images.

iii) Performance evaluation of proposed U-net based deep learning segmentation model for accurate detection of brain tumors and its performance comparison with existing (k-means and fuzzy c-means clustering) algorithms.

iv) Precise brain tumor subregions (Whole, Core, and Enhancing Tumors) analysis using the proposed deep learning models.

1.3 Literature survey

To fulfill the objectives of this thesis, clear understanding of the concept of human brain tumors, image processing, and machine learning are necessary. For this purpose, several books like John L Semmlow, 2004; Rafael C. Gonzales, 2008; Ingo Steinwart and Andreas Christann, 2003; Jayaramans., et al., 2009; William K. Pratt, 2001; Ian Goodfellow,et al., 2016; François Chollet, 2017 are studied.

1.3.1 Research gaps

Despite recent developments in semi-automatic and fully automatic algorithms for MRI brain tumor segmentation and classification, there are still several challenges for this task mainly due to the high variation of brain tumors in size, shape, regularity, location, and their heterogeneous appearance. After completion of literature survey in the brain tumor segmentation area, the following research gaps are observed: i) The Brain Blood Blurry (BBB) normally remains intact in Low Grade Glioma (LGG) cases and the tumor regions are usually not contrast-enhanced; therefore, the boundaries of LGG can be invisible or blurry despite Fluid Attenuate Image Recovery (FLAIR) sequence may provide differentiation between normal brain and brain tumor or edema to describe the full extent of the tumor. ii) In contrast, for High Grade Gliomas (HGG) cases, the contrast agent, e.g., gadolinium, leaks across the disrupted BBB and enters extracellular space of the brain tumor causing hyper-intensity on T1-weighted images. Therefore, the necrosis and active tumor regions can be easily delineated. However, HGG usually exhibits unclear and irregular boundaries that might also involve discontinuities due to aggressive tumor infiltration. This can cause problems and result in poor tumor segmentation. iii) Various tumor subregions and tumor types can only be visible by considering multi-modal MRI data. However, the co-registration across multiple MRI sequences can be difficult especially when these sequences are acquired in different spatial resolutions. iv) Typical clinical MR images are normally acquired with higher in-plane resolution and much lower inter-slice resolution. This is to balance between adequate image slices to cover the whole tumor volume with good quality cross-sectional views and the restricted scanning time.

In this research, with consideration of above research challenges, an automatic detection, classification and extraction of subregions of brain tumor MRI is performed for better diagnose of disease.

Literature study on denoising of Brain Tumor images

Medical imaging modalities include Computed Tomography (CT), Positron Emission Tomography (PET), Single Photon Emission Computed Tomography (SPECT) and Magnetic Resonance Imaging (MRI) scanners. In addition to these, many scanning techniques have been used to see the physical body for diagnostic and treatment purposes. Also, these modalities are very useful for patient follow-up, with regards to the progress of the disease state, when already been diagnosed. The overwhelming majority of imaging is predicated on the appliance of X-rays and ultrasound. These medical imaging modalities are involved altogether level of hospitalization. Additionally, they are instrumental within the public health and medicine settings also as within the curative and further extending to palliative care. The main objective is to determine the right diagnoses.

Cihangiroglu M R et al., (2003) have analyzed over 20,000 imaging studies of CT, MRI, SPECT, and PET modalities in traumatic brain injury. Saptalaka B.K., and Rajeshwari (2013) have presented a survey about MRI techniques. To visualize the information of various tissues of the human body, MRI is typically used in radiology. As it offers greater contrast between the diverse soft tissues of the body than the CT, it is useful in neurological and oncological imaging. MRI uses an effective magnetic field to line up the nuclear magnetization of hydrogen atoms in water in the body as it does not use ionizing radiation and is however different from CT.

F. Seggone et al., (2014), have displayed a novel skull-stripping calculation in light of a mixed approach that joins watershed calculations and deformable surface models. In that strategy, it takes the value of the robustness and in addition the surface data accessible to the last mentioned. In the calculation essential concentration is a single white issue voxel in a T1-weighted MR image, and uses it to make a global minimum in the white issue before applying a watershed calculation with a pre flooding stature.

Filtering methods are generally preferred for reducing noise in an image. Gaussian noise is evenly distributed over the image and has a normal Gaussian distribution function. Salt and pepper noise has white and black pixels corresponding to the minimum and maximum values. Speckle noise mostly occurs in medical images as a multiplicative noise and has gamma distribution. Poisson noise is defined as the root mean square value and the noises at different pixels are independent of one another which is proportional to the square root of the image intensity. Poisson noise has Poisson distribution and approximates to Gaussian noise other than very low-intensity levels. In image denoising, discriminative learning methods have been widely considered due to its good performance and fast inference. However, for denoising images with different noise levels needs multiple models and these methods mostly learn a specific model for each noise level.

Zhang et al., (2017) have proposed feed-forward denoising CNNs (DnCNNs) and also introduced residual learning and batch standardization into image denoising for the first time. For noisy images, the parameters are trained using a fixed variance σ. The model uses a residual learning function to study a mapping function and to accelerate the training procedure it combines it with batch normalization to improve the denoising results. The integration of residual learning and batch normalization can benefit each other and it turns out to be effective in speeding up the training and boosting denoising performance but the trained model under σ is not suitable for other noise variances. With an unknown noise level, the denoising method enables the user to adaptively make a trade-off between texture protection and noise suppression.

Zhang et al., (2018) introduced a Fast and Flexible Denoising Convolutional Neural Network (FFDNet). The FFDNet worked on down sampled sub images, attaining a good trade-off between denoising performance and inference speeds. The

7

FFDNet has the following capabilities: i) Effectively handles an extensive range of noise levels with a single network; ii) removes spatially variant noise by defining a non-uniform noise level map; and ii) quicker speed than benchmark BM3D (Hasan M and M R El-Sakka, 2018) without sacrificing denoising performance. Even though BM3D attains good denoising performance, when images are contaminated by huge noise levels it is not sufficient to denoise the images.

Nanthagopal P et al., (2013) discussed the elimination of non-brain tissue which are the major requirement for MS analysis and tumor segmentation in MR brain images and focused on 2-Dimensional Discrete Wavelet Transform (2D-DWT). Noise removal is carried out using 2D-DWT and found that diversities and ambiguous boundaries limit the classification performance. Rosniza Roslan et al., (2011) have presented the method called region developing and numerical morphology for skull stripping. The quality and limitations of these two strategies have been explored in this system on three sorts of MRI brain pictures. Their skull stripping comes about more vigorous and precise contrasted with other regular strategies.

Gonzales and Woods (2002) have characterized scientific morphology for extracting picture parts like skull and are supportive in the portrayal and depiction of different shape, for instance, limits, skeletons, and arched structure. To deal with various issues of preparing picture it provides a straightforward and productive path for coordinating separation, neighborhood data as the morphological operation requires double frame pictures in division and carried together in an intense way. Morphology needs an earlier binarization of the image. Abdulaziz Saleh et al., (2016) have presented to remove the speckle noise using mean, median and adaptive median filter from medical images and performance of the filters are compared. Deepa P. and Suganthi M. (2014) have suggested linear and nonlinear filtering techniques that are useful for medical images. Image degradation of these techniques have investigated the performance problem which may happen during the acquisition of images, optical effects such as blurring out of focus, flat-bed scanner, and camera motion. The performance of these techniques are evaluated in terms of PSNR and MSE.

Dimitri V D Ville et al., (2003) have proposed a new method for fuzzy filtering. The method first decreases the adaptive noise and then smoothing in the second stage is carried out by the fuzzy derivation for the image. Jinshan Tang (2009) have proposed a new filter called Anistropic Diffusion (AD) which is robust to noise and then multi direction Gradient Vector Flow (GVF) is used for segmentation which segments skin cancer region traces even in the presence of other skin region.

Literature study on classification of Brain Tumors

Classification and clustering methods are composed mainly by machine learning algorithms. Machine learning provides an effective way to automate the analysis and diagnosis for medical images. It can potentially reduce the burden on radiologists in the practice of radiology, which can learn complex relationships or patterns from empirical data and make accurate decisions. Machine learning algorithms can be organized into different categories based on different principles.

The classification is categorized into supervised learning, semi-supervised learning, and unsupervised learning algorithms based on the utilization of labels of training samples. In fact, most of brain tumor segmentation algorithms are based on classification or clustering methods in the literature such as Fuzzy C-Means (FCM), k-means, Artificial Neural Networks (ANN), and Support Vector Machines (SVM), etc. Deep learning methods present an improvement over non-deep learning methods. However, Support Vector Machine (SVM) and Neural Networks (NN) are the widely used approaches for their good performance over the last few decades. But recently, deep learning models set an exciting trend in machine learning as the deep architecture can efficiently represent complex relationships without requiring a huge number of nodes like in the shallow architectures e.g., SVM and K-Nearest Neighbor (KNN).

Sachdeva et al., (2011) have proposed a new hybrid machine learning system based on the Genetic Algorithm (GA) and SVM for brain tumor classification. Texture and intensity features of tumors are taken as input. Genetic algorithm has been used to select the set of most informative input features. The study is performed on real 428 post contrast T1-weighted MR images of 55 patients. Primary brain tumors such as Astrocytoma (AS), Glioblastoma Multiforme (GBM), Meningioma (MEN), and child tumor-Medulloblastoma (MED) along with secondary tumor-Metastatic (MET) are classified by GA-SVM classifier. Test results showed that the GA optimization technique has enhanced the overall accuracy of SVM from 56.3 % to

9

91.7 %. Individual class accuracies obtained are: AS-89.8 %, GBM-83.3 %, MEN-96 %, MET-91.8 %, MED-97.1 %. A comparative study with earlier methods is also done. The study reveals that GA-SVM provides more accurate results than earlier methods and is tested on more diversified dataset.

Jiang J et al., (2013) have proposed a method to construct a graph by learning the population and patient-specific feature sets of multimodal MR images and by utilizing the graph-cut to achieve a final segmentation. The probabilities of each pixel that belongs to the foreground (tumor) and the background are estimated by global and custom classifiers that are trained through learning population- and patient-specific feature sets, respectively. The proposed method is evaluated using 23 glioma image sequences, and the segmentation results are compared with other approaches. The encouraging evaluation results obtained, i.e., DSC (84.5 %), Jaccard (74.1 %), sensitivity (87.2 %), and specificity (83.1 %), show that the proposed method can effectively make use of both population and patient-specific information.

Heba M et al., (2017) discussed an efficient methodology which combines the discrete wavelet transform (DWT) with the Deep Neural Network (DNN) to classify the brain MRIs into Normal and 3 types of malignant brain tumors: glioblastoma, sarcoma, and metastatic bronchogenic carcinoma. The new methodology architecture resembles the convolutional neural networks architecture, but requires less hardware specifications and takes a convenient time of processing for large size images. Yan Xu et al., (2015) introduced deep convolutional activation features trained to histopathology image classification and histopathology image segmentation with relatively little training data. CNN features are more powerful than manual features (an improvement of 20 points in both classification and segmentation) and due to the large size of histopathology images, feature pooling is used for a single feature vector for classification method. It achieved a-state-of-the-art accuracy of 97.5 % for classification and 84 % for segmentation of brain tumor in the MR image.

Renhao Liua et al., (2015) explored the feasibility of using a pretrained CNN as a feature extractor to get deep feature representations for brain tumor MR images. The deep features enable classifiers to have comparable or better predictive power (95 % accuracy) than conventional handcrafted feature extraction methods. From one or two features an accuracy of 90.91 % was obtained from pretreatment images showing promise for differential treatment. Tianjiao Liu et al., (2017) discussed a feature extraction method for the thyroid nodules classification. Both traditional low-level features and high-level deep features extracted from CNN model are used to provide more generic semantic meanings to the limited medical dataset. This method outperforms both the pre-trained CNN model and the traditional single-type feature method.

Shreyansh A P et al., (2017) has performed Dental disease classification using CNN with transfer learning. The common diseases like dental caries, periapical infection and periodontitis are classified as three different models on two different architectures. Transfer learning with VGG16 pretrained model is used with small dataset of 251 RVG (Radio Visio Graphy) X-ray images for training and testing purposes to achieve an overall accuracy of 88.46 %. Kaoutar B et al., (2017) has performed survival time prediction with large datasets to train complex models for transferring features of a previously trained model by fine-tuning to the new task. Deep convolutional features from raw MRI scans of different sequences based on a pretrained deep CNN features were extracted as the outputs of the final hidden layer. Symmetric uncertainty was used to select 7 features for a random forests classifier. A predictive accuracy of 81.8 % is achieved using the Flair sequence.

Imon Banerjee et al., (2018) developed an efficient CAD system for the differential diagnosis of embryonal (ERMS) and alveolar (ARMS) subtypes of Rhabdomysarcoma (RMS). The system executes a completely automatic pipeline that performs segmentation and fusion of Diffusion-Weighted MR scans (DWI) and gadolinium chelate-enhanced T1-weighted MR scans (MRI) and classifies the fused images based on a trained deep CNN model. The system derives the final patient-level diagnosis by majority voting of the fused images. Required human interaction is only limited to the manual outlining of the tumor on a single slice. System is exposited to provide a fast and reproducible diagnosis of RMS subtypes only by analyzing non-invasive multiparametric MR scans. Muhammed Talo et al., (2019) employed a popular pre-trained deep learning CNN architecture (ResNet34) to classify normal and abnormal brain MR images. To optimize hyper parameters using data augmentation technique is employed in deep learning. The developed model can be used to find other brain abnormalities like Alzheimer's disease, stroke, Parkinson's disease, and autism.

E I Zacharaki et al., 2009 has investigated the use of pattern classification methods for distinguishing different types of brain tumors, such as primary gliomas from metastases, and also for grading of gliomas. Feature subset selection is performed using SVM with recursive feature elimination. The method was applied on a population of 102 brain tumors histologically diagnosed as metastasis (24), meningiomas (4), gliomas World Health Organization grade II (22), gliomas World Health Organization grade III (18), and glioblastomas (34). The binary support vector machine classification accuracy, sensitivity, and specificity, assessed by leave-one-out cross-validation, were, respectively, 85 %, 87 %, and 79 % for discrimination of metastases from gliomas and 88 %, 85 %, and 96 % for discrimination of high-grade (grades III and IV) from low-grade (grade II) neoplasms. Abiwinanda Nyoman et al., (2019) have attempted to train a Convolutional Neural Network (CNN) to recognize the three most common types of brain tumors, i.e., the Glioma, Meningioma, and Pituitary. We implemented the simplest possible architecture of CNN; i.e. one each of convolution, max-pooling, and flattening layers, followed by a full connection from one hidden layer. The CNN was trained on a brain tumor dataset consisting of 3064 T-1 weighted CE-MR images publicly available via figshare Cheng (Brain Tumor Dataset, 2017). Using our simple architecture and without any prior region-based segmentation, the training accuracy of 98.51% and validation accuracy of 84.19 % are achieved. These figures are comparable to the performance of more complicated region-based segmentation algorithms, which accuracies ranged between 71.39 % and 94.68 % on identical dataset Cheng (Brain Tumor Dataset, 2017, Cheng et al. (PLoS One 11, 2017).

Seetha J. and S Selvakumar Raja (2018) have proposed a CNN classification based an automatic brain tumor detection. The deeper architecture design is performed by using small kernels. The weight of the neuron is given as small. Experimental results show that the CNN achieves an accuracy of 97.5 % with low complexity and compared with the all other state of arts methods.

Dou Qi et al., (2016) have proposed a novel automatic method to detect Cerebral Micro Bleeds (CMB) from MR images by exploiting the 3D CNN. To further improve the detection performance while reducing the computational cost, a cascaded framework under 3D CNNs for the task of CMB detection is proposed. Compared with traditional sliding window strategy, the proposed 3D FCN strategy can remove massive redundant computations and dramatically speed up the detection process. A large dataset with 320 volumetric MR scans was constructed and performed extensive experiments to validate the proposed method, which achieved a high sensitivity of 93.16 % with an average number of 2.74 false positives per subject, outperforming previous methods using low-level descriptors or 2D CNNs by a significant margin.

Amin Javeria et al., (2018) have proposed a methodology to segment and classify the brain tumor MRI. Deep Neural Networks (DNNs) based architecture is employed for tumor segmentation. In the proposed model, 7 layers are used for classification that consist of 3 convolutional, 3 ReLU and a softmax layer. First the input MR image is divided into multiple patches and then the center pixel value of each patch is supplied to the DNN. DNN assigns labels according to center pixels and perform segmentation. Extensive experiments are performed using eight large scale benchmark datasets including BraTS 2012 (image dataset and synthetic dataset), 2013 (image dataset and synthetic dataset), 2014, 2015 and ISLES (Ischemic stroke lesion segmentation) 2015 and 2017. The results are validated on accuracy (ACC), sensitivity (SE), specificity (SP), Dice Similarity Coefficient (DSC), precision, false positive rate (FPR), true positive rate (TPR), and Jaccard similarity Coefficient (JSC) respectively.

Swati Zar Nawab Khan et al., (2019) have used a pre-trained deep convolutional neural network model and propose a block-wise fine-tuning strategy based on transfer learning. The proposed method is evaluated on T1-weighted contrast-enhanced magnetic resonance images (CE-MRI) benchmark dataset. Our method is more generic as it does not use any handcrafted features, requires minimal preprocessing and can achieve average accuracy of 94.82 % under five-fold cross-validation. The experimental results are not only compared with the traditional machine learning but also with deep learning methods. Experimental results show that the proposed method outperforms state-of-the-art classification on the CE-MRI dataset.

13

Literature study on Brain Tumor Segmentation

Ajala Funmilola A et al., (2012) have clarified numerous methodologies used for medical image segmentation like cluster, thresholding, classifier, region growing, separate Model and so forth. Their work is particularly focused on cluster techniques, particularly k-means and fuzzy c-means cluster algorithms. They merge these equations along to make another procedure known as fuzzy k-means and fuzzy c-means group calculation. The calculations are implemented and tried with MR image of brain tumor. Results are dissected and recorded. Sezgin Mehrnet. Et al., (2004) have exhibited another image thresholding strategy in light of the divergence function. In this strategy, the objective, function is assembled utilizing the uniqueness work between the classes, the object and the foundation. The required threshold is built up where this divergence work shows a global minimum.

Islam Atiq et al., (2013) have proposed multifractal feature-based tumor segmentation. The combination of multifractal features with the Gabor-like multiscale texture features are extended in the traditional Adaboost algorithm. By this method classification accuracy is improved. Simultaneous clustering and texture feature extraction consume more time. Sudre Carole H. et al., (2015) have presented white matter lesion segmentation according to the Bayesian Model of input structure. Here, this proposed texture based Pathological Neuroimaging Data analysis is used to classify the white matter region from overall MR image. Here, they provide Bayesian model selection with gradient approach of image feature analysis and segmentation of white Matter. This can be done with edge based feature identification. Segmentation rate for Bayesian method is raised up to the average value of 90 %. In this texture extraction if there is any intensity variation in the image, then it misclassifies as tumor spot. This increase the time complexity due to the increase in image feature.

Anitha V and S Murugavalli (2016) have projected system practices the adaptive pillar k-means algorithm which performs the effective segmentation and the classification by means of the two-tier classification method. The proposed novel two-tier classification system improves the classification accuracy by means of brain tumors in double training procedure and the performances are compared with the other traditional classification technique in relations of the performance procedures such as sensitivity, specificity, and classification accuracy. Results specified that the

14

projected novel two class classifier generates greater improvement in performance when related with SVM based classification system.

Nasibov E N and G Ulutagay (2007) have introduced Fuzzy Joint Points (FJP) for the purpose of initial clusters, cluster validity and direct clustering. Barakbah A R, and Y Kiyoki (2009) have presented Pillar k-means algorithm to optimize k-means clustering. The space among all the centroids and all the new data points have been determined. Then new data points which have maximum distance have been selected as new centroid point. The number of features used for classification is reduced by PCA and LDA methods. The SVM classifier is served as an evaluation of nonlinear techniques and linear ones. Ahmed Mohamed N. et al., (2002) have exhibited a creative strategy for modified fuzzy c-means calculation in distinguishing the target capacity of standard fuzzy c-means calculation. This is helpful for brain MRI influenced by salt and pepper combination of examining machine.

Cuadra et al., (2004) have proposed a technique to deform brain atlas within the existence of huge space-occupying tumors, supported a priori model of lesion advance by assuming that the lesion expands from the starting point. Ronneberger et al., (2015) have suggested a network and string that is in agreement with the effective use of deep networks using data augmentation to make more efficient use of the available labeled samples. Işın Ali et al., (2016) have given an impression of all MRI brain tumor segmentation using DL techniques and explains how these methods give far superior results compared to traditional methods in terms of effective processing and evaluation of large input image data. Sergio Pereira et al., (2016) proposed a reliable and automatic segmentation technique supported CNN; which explores small 3x3 filters due to deeper architecture, and utilized normalization of intensity as pre-processing step together with augmentation of data and proved to be very effective.

Hao Dong et al., (2017) suggested, and assessed on BraTS 2015 datasets, a reliable and fully automatic segmentation technique using U-Net-based FCN for effective tumor measurement. Cross-validation has demonstrated that their technique effectively delivers promising segmentation results. M. Havaei et al., (2017) have suggested a fully automatic brain tumor segmentation technique specifically designed for low and high grade MR image glioblastomas using a novel CNN architecture with

15

a fully connected layer, allowing 40-fold speed and a double stage training procedure that enables tumor label imbalance challenges to be addressed. In the 2013 BraTS, a cascade of CNNs was also used to achieve higher data rates. Kamnitsas et al., (2017) suggested a dual, 11-layer deep, 3D CNN network to divide the brain lesion resulting from a thorough assessment of current network constraints.

Qingneng Li, et al., (2018) have proposed an automatic glioma segmentation algorithm by first using spatial fuzzy c-means clustering to estimate ROI in multimodal MR brain tumor images, and a few seed points are extracted from there to use region growing supported algorithm on a replacement affinity. High metric values of Dice, Sensitivity, Positive Predictive Value (PPV), Euclidean distance (ED), and Hausdorff distance (HD) are obtained with rank of number one when obtained performance metrics compared with the state-of-the-art methods. Andriy Myronenko (2018) has proposed an automated segmentation of volumetric MR brain tumor images which is required to diagnose, monitor, and treatment planning of the disease. They described semantic segmentation model based on encoder-decoder architecture for extracting the tumor sub-region from 3D MRIs and won first place in the 2018 BraTS challenge.

Sajid Iqbal et al., (2018) presented an extended version of multiple neural network layers connected to peer-level feeding of Convolutional feature maps in sequential order for segmentation of brain tumor in multi-spectral MRI using CNN on BraTS dataset. Fabian Isensee et al., (2018) has shown the adequacy of a well-trained U-Net with regard to the BraTS 2018 challenge which improved the segmentation performance with minor adjustments in the network design. A large patch size was used to make the training dataset and the proposed network was trained with the above dataset using a dice loss function. An aggressive Dice scores are accomplished on validation data and stood in second position. Raghav Mehta et al., (2018) presented Multimodal brain MR volumes with a 3D CNN for segmentation of brain tumor by using a 3D U-net modified design. The adjustment here is a stronger gradient flow, which helps the network to learn learnable parameters effectively and to produce better segmentation. 2018 BraTS training dataset is used to train the network and good segmentation results are obtained.

Jean Stawiaski (2018) has presented a DenseNet based on a densely connected convolution network encoder for automatic segmentation of MRI brain tumor in 3D multi-modal images and attained the average DSC scores of 0.79, 0.90, and 0.85 for ET, WT, and TC, respectively, by evaluating the challenge of BraTS 2018. Xue Feng et al., (2018) suggested a 3D U-net for segmentation of MRI brain tumor with diverse hyper parameters and a linear model is developed from extracted features of imaging and non-imaging for patient survival prediction. The average dice scores of 0.7917, 0.9094, and 0.8362 are achieved for ET, WT, and TC, respectively. Richard McKinley et al., (2018) launched a novel classifier family using DeepSCAN architecture in which tightly linked dilated convolution blocks are integrated in a shallow down or up-sampling U-net-style connection framework. These networks are trained using the 2018 database of the Multimodal BraTS.

Tiejun Yang et al., (2019) proposed a deep learning system combining small kernels two path CNN (SK-TPNN) and random forest algorithm for the segmentation of brain tumors in MRI. The SK-TPCNN structure combines small convolution kernels with large convolution kernels to improve the capacity of nonlinear mapping and prevents over-fitting, and also increases the multiformity of features. The algorithm is validated and evaluated on the BraTS challenge of 2015. Kai Hu et al., (2019) suggested a novel technique based on multi-cascaded CNN (MCCNN) and FC (Fully Connected) conditional random fields (CRFs) for brain tumor segmentation. They trained three models for segmentation using image patches obtained from three different orientations like sagittal, coronal, and axial; and final result is obtained by combining them all.

1.4 Technical Approach

The main objective of this thesis is to assist the radiologist for a proper planning of treatment by analyzing the multimodal MR images of brain tumor to detect the tumor size, location, and shape precisely. Then the radiologist or a doctor can take consistent decisions and plan for the best possible treatment, so that the patient's survival rate can be improved. This thesis focuses on MRI brain tumor image noise reduction techniques, classification, and segmentation of MRI brain tumor subregions based on deep learning models.

During transmission or acquisition of medical images, they are degraded and mostly corrupted by Gaussian and speckle noises in addition to salt and pepper, poisson noises. These noises are removed using various filtering techniques without affecting the image quality. Denoising is an essential preprocessing task performed for medical images before classification and segmentation. Images considered for denoising task are corrupted in three ways. Firstly, image is corrupted by adding gaussian noise with wide range of noise level from 5 to 50. Second, image is corrupted by adding speckle noise with wide range of noise level from 5 to 50. Third, image is corrupted by adding different noises like Gaussian, salt and pepper, poisson, and speckle noise with a specified noise level of 15.

Generally, traditional filters (Gaussian, Guided, Adaptive, and Bilateral) are used for denoising purpose, but they suffer from three major drawbacks: i) Involve a complex optimization problem in the testing stage, making the denoising process time consuming and hardly achieve high performance without sacrificing computational efficiency, ii) These models are nonconvex and involve several manually chosen parameters. iii) They train a specific model for a certain noise level, and are limited in blind image denoising in addition to inherently complex in structure of medical image.

To overcome these limitations, a discriminative learning method that is deep learning based models (pretrained DnCNN and proposed DeepCNN) are implemented to also get rid of the iterative optimization procedure in the test phase. The reasons for using CNN are three fold. First, CNN with very deep architecture is effective in increasing the capacity and flexibility to exploit image characteristics. Second, considerable advances have been achieved on regularization and learning methods for training CNN, including Rectifier Linear Unit (ReLU), batch normalization and residual learning. These methods can be adopted to improve denoising performance. Third, CNN is well suited for parallel computation on modern powerful GPU which can be exploited to improve the run time performance.

DnCNN is a pretrained Convolutional Neural Network (CNN) (Jain, Viren et al., 2009, Xiao-Ping Zhang, 2001) used for image denoising purpose. The DnCNN (Zhang, Kai et al., 2017, K. Simonyan et al., 2015) is a 20 convolutional layer depth pretrained model for performing image denoising task and contains a total of 59 layers including one input layer, 20 convolutional layers, 19 ReLU layers, 18 batch normalization layers, and one regression output layer. The DnCNN is a well trained model on millions of natural images database set called ImageNet and these optimized weights are used to reduce the noise.

To improve the denoising performance, the network has to be trained with our data images and to achieve this, a deep learning model DeepCNN is proposed. As the pretrained DnCNN network does not offer much flexibility on the type of noise recognized since the network or model is directly considered here with a limited range of noise level without training on our data images. The proposed DeepCNN model contains a total of 50 layers including one input layer, 17 convolutional layers, 16 ReLU layers, 15 batch normalization layers, and one regression output layer. An image of patch size 50 pixels × 50 pixels is used with DnCNN whereas 61 pixels × 61 pixels is used in DeepCNN for input layers. Due to batch normalization, ReLU, and 17 convolutional layers, the training process gets speeded up, boosts the denoising performance and over fitting problem is also avoided by doing augmentation of the datasets. So, the proposed DeepCNN method gives better performance in achieving denoising task better than other methods. BraTS 2018 database is considered to prepare the image datastore size of 400 images and used for training this DeepCNN model. The results of proposed DeepCNN model is compared with DnCNN and the proposed DeepCNN model has achieved superior PSNR, SSIM, MSE, and MAE in terms of performance metrics.

The classification task is performed after denoising to classify the MR brain tumor images into either LGG or HGG using transfer learning and hybrid methods. For Transfer Learning, AlexNet architecture is considered as a pretrained model and the last few layers of the pretrained model are tuned for two class (LGG and HGG) classification problem. The learnable parameters (weights and biases) are updated to minimize the loss function using either ADAM or SGDM optimizer. The hybrid models are proposed based on the advantages of high level complex representative features extracted using CNN model and then combined with shallow machine learning algorithms like k-Nearest Neighbors (KNN) Discriminant (DISCR), Support Vector Machine (SVM), Naive Bayes (NB), Ensemble (ENSEMBLE), and Decision Tree (TREE). Various hybrid models for classification are CNN-KNN, CNN-DISCR,

CNN-SVM, CNN-NB, and CNN-ENSEMBLE. Experiments are conducted on open dataset images chosen from BraTS 2018 for classification and the proposed transfer learning with ADAM optimizer is proven to be better in terms of accuracy, error rate, F1-score, sensitivity, and specificity on the test set.

The models used for automatic segmentation are k-means, fuzzy c-means clustering algorithms and proposed DL models. The proposed DL models are constructed on the basis of U-net and VGG16 model architectures. The brain tumor subregions segmentation process consists of two DL models. First, a 23 layer DL model is used to segment full tumor (whole tumor). Second, then the segmentation results are used as input to two 18 layer DL models and combined with T1c image modality to segment the whole tumor into enhancing tumor and tumor core. To obtain the 18 layer proposed DL model, C4 block from contracting path and E1 block from expanding path are removed (Fig. 5.4). The whole tumor is obtained mainly by segmenting the T2-weighted images and is used to cross check the edema's extension in FLAIR (Fluid Attenuated Inversion Recovery) image. Enhancing Tumor (ET) and Tumor Core (TC) are both extracted by evaluating the hyper-intensities in T1-weighted contrast enhanced images. The proposed models are trained on BraTS 2018 database, evaluated on HGG cases and compared each other with performance evaluation metrics like accuracy, error rate, sensitivity, specificity, F1-measure, dice similarity coefficient, and jaccard similarity coefficient.

1.5 Applications of the thesis

The algorithms developed and analysis of work carried out in this thesis are useful for identifying the brain tumor sub regions accurately, so that patient's survival rate can be improved.

i) Implementation of DeepCNN based denoising procedure prior to classification and segmentation, the accuracy of classification and segmentation is improved and this helps in identification of brain tumor precisely.

ii) Transfer learning and hybrid models based classification methods developed in this thesis helps the radiologist to treat the cancerous tumor case for better diagnosis.

iii) Segmentation analysis of tumor based on the size, location, and shape, of tumor is not only assessing the severity of the tumor and also useful to the radiologist to avoid injury to other healthy parts during the therapy.

iv) Precise extraction methods of subregions of a brain tumor presented in this thesis are useful in the improvement of patient's survival rate.

1.6 Organization of the thesis

This thesis is organized into six chapters including Introduction and Conclusions. **Chapter 2** describes the introduction of brain tumors, different MRI modalities and the datasets used for evaluation purpose. The denoising of MR brain tumor images using traditional filters and proposed deep learning models are discussed in **chapter 3**. **Chapter 4** presents performance evaluation of proposed transfer learning model and hybrid models for classification of brain tumors. **Chapter 5** presents the proposed deep learning models for precise extraction of brain tumor and its subrerions. The overall conclusions of the thesis along with the scope for the further work are provided in **Chapter 6**.

Chapter 2

Introduction to Brain Tumor and Database

2.1 Introduction

A tumor is an abnormal growth of cells (Buehring G C and R R Williams, 1976) in the body and is broadly grouped into two classes: benign and malignant. Irrespective of its type, the tumors can develop inside the brain tissue itself (primary), or cancer from somewhere else in the body can spread to the brain (metastasis). Decision for treatment changes relying upon the tumor type, size, and location. Treatment objectives might be remedial or can even concentrate on easing symptoms. By identifying the tumors at an earlier stage, nearly 120 types of such cases are successfully treated and still striving to improve the life span of many people by introducing new therapies. This chapter is organized as follows. Section 2.2 presents an overview of brain tumors types, causes, symptoms, and statistics of brain tumors. Various orientations, modalities of MRI, and tumor subregions are explained in section 2.3. BraTS database is discussed briefly in section 2.4. Finally, conclusions are given in section 2.5.

2.2 Brain tumors

Normal cells in a body grow in a controlled way while the new cells replace old or damaged ones, whereas tumor cells reproduce uncontrollably and are not replaced with new cells. A tumor which grows in brain is called brain tumor and is shown in the Fig. 2.1.

A primary brain tumor (Surawicz T S et al., 1999) is an abnormal growth that starts in the brain and it does not generally spread to other parts of the body. They can be classified into either benign or malignant. The growth of a benign brain tumor is slow, has distinct boundaries, and it rarely spreads. But the benign tumors can be life threatening if they are located in a vital area.

22

A malignant brain tumor grows quickly, has irregular boundaries, and spreads to nearby brain areas. They are often called brain cancer, but malignant brain tumors do not fit the definition of cancer as the organs outside the brain and spine are not affected by them.

The metastatic (secondary) brain tumors (Weidle U H et al., 2015) begin as cancer somewhere else in the body and spread to the brain. They form when cancer cells are carried in the blood stream. The lung and breast cancers are the most common cancers that spread to the brain.

Primary (benign or malignant), or secondary (metastatic) brain tumors are potentially life-threatening. The brain cannot expand to make room for a growing mass as it is enclosed within the bony skull. And as a result, the tumor compresses and normal brain tissue is displaced by it. Some brain tumors cause a blockage of cerebrospinal fluid (CSF) (Linninger A et al., 2007) that flows around and through the brain which increases intracranial pressure and ventricles (hydrocephalus) can be enlarged by this. Some brain tumors cause swelling (edema) (Unterberg A W et al., 2004). Size, pressure, and swelling all create mass effect, which cause many of the symptoms. They may also grow from the brain tissue itself (glioma) (Giesexs A and M Westphal, 1996). As they grow they may compress normal tissue and cause symptoms.

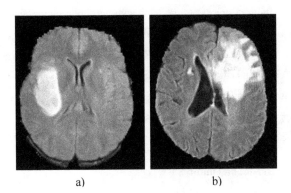

a)   b)

Fig. 2.1 Brain tumors of MR images. a) LGG (benign) image

b) HGG (malignant) image.

2.2.1 Types of brain tumors

A classification and grading system was developed by the World Health Organization (WHO) to standardize communication, treatment planning, and in predicting the outcomes for brain tumors. The tumors can be classified based on the cell type and grade by viewing the cells, usually taken during a biopsy, under a microscope.

2.2.1.1 Cell type

It refers to the cell of origin of the tumor. For example, nerve cells (neurons) and support cells (glial and schwann cells) give rise to tumors. About half of all primary brain tumors grow from glial cells (gliomas) (Silbergeld D L and M R Chicoine, 1997). There are many types of gliomas because there are different kinds of glial cells.

Glial cells are supportive tissues of brain and classified into four types:
- i. Astrocytes-These are blood brain barriers.
- ii. Oligodendrocytes-These produce covering (myelin) to neurons.
- iii. Microglia-These destroy pathogens that invade brain and similar are to white blood cells.
- iv. Ependymal cells-These align the ventricles and secrete cerebrospinal fluid.

Gliomas tumors are the most common brain tumors that emerge from glial of the brain. According to BraTS database the gliomas tumors are characterized into two types: LGG and HGG. The LGG case consists of grade I and grade II tumors. Generally, LGG cases exhibit benign tendencies and a very less number of LGG cases exhibit malignant tendencies. The HGG case consists of grade III and grade IV tumors. These are malignant tumors and having more aggressiveness. These grades will be discussed in the next section.

2.2.1.2 Grades of Tumor

Brain tumors are categorized in the medical field by their grade. The grade of a tumor is decided as per the behavior under microscopic observation:

GRADE I: These tumors are known as benign which appear same as normal brain cells but they have slow growth rate in comparison with other grades. This is the first stage of tumor. The characteristics include slow growing cells, almost normal appearance, least malignant, usually associated with long-term survival.

GRADE II: These tumors having less malignant tendencies. Grade I and Grade II are known as low grade tumors. The characteristics include relatively slow growing cells, slightly abnormal appearance, nearby tissue can be invaded, and sometimes recur as a higher grade.

GRADE III: They require urgent treatment to cure and behave differently from normal cells. The characteristics include actively reproducing abnormal cells, abnormal appearance, infiltrate normal tissue, tend to recur, often as a higher grade.

GRADE IV: The fastest growth rate types of tumors are grade IV and have abnormal behavior than other grades. Grade III and Grade IV are known as high grade tumors. The characteristics include rapidly reproducing abnormal cells, very abnormal appearance, area of dead cells (necrosis) in center, and form new blood vessels to maintain growth.

Grade of tumor denotes the manner in which tumor cells look under the microscope and is an indication of aggressiveness. The tumors often have a mix of cell grades and can change as they grow. Differentiated and anaplastic are terms used to describe how similar or abnormal the tumor cells appear compared to normal cells.

The growth of a tumor from stage I to stage IV depends on age and immunity system of the patient, environment where the patent is living, genetic and biological nature of the patient.

2.2.2 Causes of brain tumors

Medical science neither knows what causes brain tumors nor how to prevent primary tumors that start in the brain. People who are at risk from brain tumors include those who have: Cancer elsewhere in the body, prolonged exposure to pesticides, industrial solvents, and other chemicals, and inherited diseases such as neurofibromatosis.

2.2.3 Symptoms of brain tumors

Tumors can affect the brain by destroying normal tissue, compressing normal tissue or increasing intracranial pressure. Symptoms vary depending on the tumor's type, size, and location in the brain. The general symptoms include, headaches that tend to worsen in the morning, seizures, stumbling, dizziness, difficulty in walking, speech problems (e.g., difficulty finding the right word), vision problems, abnormal eye movements, weakness on one side of the body, increased intracranial pressure which causes drowsiness, headaches, nausea and vomiting, sluggish responses.

2.2.4 Statistics on brain tumors

The gliomas brain tumors comprises of 80.7 % of all malignant tumors (Wang, Qing et al., 2019) and 26.5 % of all primary brain tumors. In 2018 itself, there are around 80,000 new malignant cases and nonmalignant primary brain tumor and other CNS (Central Nervous System) tumors were reported to be diagnosed. Among them, around 32 % are reported to have primary malignant tumors and other CNS tumors. Also, there are around 17,000 deaths reported during the year 2018 due to the same problem. Only 34.9 % of 5 year relative survival rate has been reported after being diagnosed with primary malignant brain and other CNS tumors and it is only 90.47 % for the cases with primary nonmalignant brain tumors (Ostrom Quinn T et al., 2019). Although brain tumors can occur at any age, they are most common in children 3 to 12 years old and in adults 40 to 70 years old.

2.3 Medical brain imaging

The commonly available brain imaging techniques for diagnosis are Computed Tomography (CT) (Bilaniuk L T et al., 1980), Positron Emission Tomography (PET) (Bergsneider M et al., 1997), Single Photon Emission Computed Tomography (SPECT) (Holly T A et al., 2010) and Magnetic Resonance Imaging (MRI) (Liang Z P and P C Lauterbur, 2000). The most popular imaging technique is MRI which provide the exact information about tumor and its subregions.

Magnetic field and radio frequency waves are used by the MRI scan to give a thorough picture of the soft tissues of the brain. It views the brain 3-dimensionally in slices that can be taken from the side or from the top as a cross-section by injecting a dye into the bloodstream. It is very useful to evaluate brain lesions and their effects on surrounding brain. Brain tumor of MR images are acquired in three orientations and four modalities. The images acquired have the orientation of Axial, Sagittal, and Coronal as shown in Fig. 2.2.

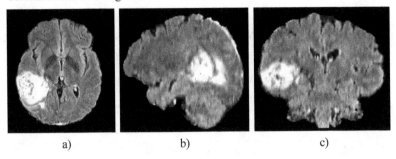

a)   b)   c)

Fig. 2.2 Various orientations of MRI sequence modalities. a) Axial b) Sagittal c) Coronal.

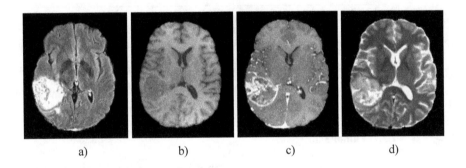

a)   b)   c)   d)

Fig. 2.3 MRI sequence modalities. a) Fluid Attenuated Inversion Recovery (FLAIR) image b) T1-weighted image c) T1-Contrast enhancement (T1Gad or T1c) image d) T2-weighted image.

Each orientation of the MR image is described as T1-weighted native image (T1), T1-weighted image post-contrast enhancement (T1c), T2-weighted native image (T2), and T2 weighted FLAIR (Fluid Attenuated Inversion Recovery) image as shown in below Fig. 2.3. The differences among all the modalities are given in able 2.1. The Cerebral spinal fluid (CSF) appears as dark in T1 imaging and bright in T2 imaging. Another commonly used MRI scan sequence is the T2-weighted FLAIR which is like a T2-weighted image.

27

Abnormalities continue to be bright, however, the CSF is attenuated and created dark in FLAIR. So, it is very easy to differentiate the abnormality and CSF in FLAIR imaging. Gadolinium (Gad) is a post contrast enhancing agent in T1-weighted imaging (T1c). When it is injected throughout the MRI scan, it changes pixel intensities by shortening T1. Accordingly, Gad is very bright on T1c images. T1c images are particularly helpful in observing breakdown in the blood-brain barrier and vascular structures.

Table 2.1 Modalities of MR image.

Sl. No	Tissue	T1- weighted	T2-weighted	FLAIR
1	CSF	Dark	Bright	Dark
2	White Matter	Light	Dark Gray	Dark Gray
3	Fat	Bright	Light	Light
4	Edema (infection)	Dark	Bright	Bright

HGG (malignant) tumors have an irregular border that invades normal tissue with finger-like projections making surgical removal more difficult. LGG (Benign) tumors have relatively clear edges than HGG tumor and somewhat easily removed surgically.

2.3.1 Tumor subregions

The tumor is extracted as Enhancing Tumor (ET), Tumor Core (TC), and Whole Tumor (WT) shown in below Fig. 2.4 and Fig. 2.5. The ET is indicated with green color and is a part of the tumor core, which in turn is surrounded by whole tumor. Appearance of the ET leads to human life threatening i.e., most of the HGG (malignant) cases involve enhancing tumor. The tumor core is a part of the whole tumor, represented with red color and entailed by ET.

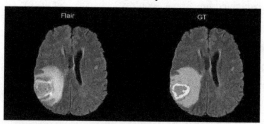

Fig. 2.4 Subregions of HGG (malignant) brain tumor of MR image.
Flair image (left), Ground truth image (right).

28

It is described as the necrotic (fluid-filled) and the nonenhancing (solid) parts of the tumor. The complete extension of the tumor is described as the whole tumor, as it entails the TC and the WT, and is indicated by green color. In LGG case, mostly the tumors do not have enhancing tumor. Examination of HGG case is more essential than that of LGG cases.

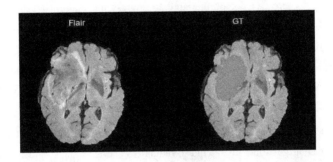

Fig. 2.5 Subregions of LGG (benign) brain tumor of MR image.
Flair image (left), Ground truth image (right).

2.4 BraTS database

The scope of the BraTS (Menze, BH. et al., 2014, Bakas, S. et al., 2017b) challenge (http://braintumorsegmentation.org) is that the specialized best segmentation techniques are used to analyze brain tumor in MRI multimodal sequence scans. The multi-institutional MRI sequence scans of pre-operative images are used in BraTS 2018 database and concentrated on segmentation of heterogeneous brain tumors, particularly gliomas, moreover, to locate the medical importance of the segmentation task.

2.4.1 Clinical relevance

The most common primary brain malignancies are the gliomas, which varies aggressively, variable diagnosis and various heterogeneous histological subregions, i.e., necrotic core, peritumoral edema, enhancing and nonenhancing tumor core. This inherent heterogeneity of gliomas is also represented in their imaging phenotype

29

(appearance and shape), as their subregions are labelled by varying intensity profiles disseminated across multimodal MRI scans, which reflects varying biological properties of a tumor. Because of the highly heterogeneous appearance and shape, segmentation of brain tumors in multimodal MRI scans is one of the most challenging tasks in medical image analysis.

There is a lot of literature to address the important task on computational algorithms. But, presently there are no open datasets for designing and testing these algorithms. The private datasets vary so extensively that it is difficult to compare the various segmentation strategies which are reported till now. The various critical factors which leads to these differences are: i) various imaging modalities that are employed, ii) the tumor type (HGG or LGG, solid or infiltratifvely growing, primary or secondary), and iii) the state of disease (images can be acquired prior to treatment as well as post-operatively and so radiotherapy effects and surgically-imposed cavities are shown). BraTS is making such a large dataset available which is accompanied with delineations of the related tumor subregions.

2.4.2 Segmentation of gliomas in pre-operative MRI scans

The labels given in the BraTS database are '1' for NET (Non Enhancing Tumor) and NCR (Necrotic), '2' for ED (Edema), '4' for ET (Enhancing Tumor) or Active Tumor (AT), 0 for everything else as shown in Fig. 2.6 (taken from BraST 2018). In this work, three glioma sub regions are used to evaluate the segmentation method which are ET, WT, and TC respectively. The Enhancing Tumor (ET) is calculated by finding the area of hyper-intensity in T1c (Litjens G et al., 2017) or T1c image when contrasted with image T1-weighted, yet additionally, when contrasted with healthy white matter in T1c image. The ET is segmented from label 4 in T1c image modality of database. The Core Tumor (CT) is segmented by using the combination of labels 1 and 4 in T1c image. The TC describes the nonenhancing and also the necrotic tumor regions. The presence of NCR and NET tumor core is regularly hypo-intense in T1c when contrasted with T1. The Whole Tumor (WT) consists of labels 1, 2, and 4 and is a complete extension of the tumor which is segmented mainly from T2 and FLAIR. It is utilized to check the edema's extension and separate it against ventricles and other necrotic structures.

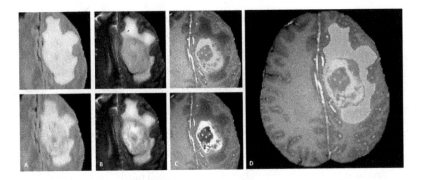

Fig. 2.6 Tumor structures present on the image patches interpreted in different modalities (top left) and the final labels for the whole dataset (right). Image patches shown (left to right): the WT visible in FLAIR (A), the tumor core visible in T2 (B), the enhancing tumor structures visible in T1c (blue), surrounding the cystic/necrotic components of the core (green) (C). Final labels of the tumor structures generated after combining the segmentations (D): edema (yellow), nonenhancing solid core (red), necrotic/cystic core (green), enhancing core (blue).

2.4.3 Imaging data description

All BraTS multimodal scans can be accessed as NIfTI files (.nii.gz) which describes a) native (T1) and b) post-contrast T1-weighted (T1Gad or T1c), c) T2-weighted (T2), and d) T2 Fluid Attenuated Inversion Recovery (FLAIR) volumes, and are acquired with various clinical protocols and different scanners from multiple institutions, also stated as data contributors.

One to four experts have manually segmented all the imaging datasets (Bakas S et al., 2017a), by using the same annotation protocol, and experienced neuro-radiologists have approved their annotations. The annotations include the Gad-enhancing tumor (ET label 4), the peritumoral edema (ED label 2), and the necrotic and nonenhancing tumor core (NCR/NET label 1). After preprocessing, the provided data is distributed, i.e. co-registered to the same anatomical template, interpolated to the same resolution (1 mm^3) and then skull-stripped.

2.4.4 Comparison with previous BraTS database

There is a significant difference between the BraTS data provided since BraTS 2017 and that was provided during the previous BraTS challenges (i.e., 2016 and backwards). The clinical experts have manually annotated the images and annotations of BraTS 2012-13, and it is the only data that have been previously used and will be utilized again (during BraTS 2017-18). The data used during BraTS 2014-16 (from TCIA) describes a mixture of pre and post-operative scans. The fusion of segmentation results from algorithms that ranked highly during BraTS 2012 and 2013 is used to annotate the ground truth labels and thus they have been discarded. In 2018, the complete original TCIA glioma collections were radiologically assessed by the expert neuro radiologists and each scan is categorized by them as pre or post-operative. Then, they have annotated all the pre-operative TCIA scans (135 GBM and 108 LGG) for the various glioma subregions and included in the BraTS datasets of the year 2018.

2.4.5 Previous BraTS challenges

BraTS is a popular database which releases MRI preprocessed labelled brain tumor images and it conducts challenge every year by updating the image database. BraTS 2018 is built upon its eight previous successful instances which are BraTS 2012 (Nice, France), BraTS 2013 (Nagoya, Japan), BraTS 2014 (Boston, USA), BraTS 2015 (Munich, Germany), BraTS 2016 (Athens, Greece), BraTS 2017 (Quebec City, Canada), BraTS 2018 (Granada, Spain), and BraTS 2019 (Shenzhen, China).

2.4.6 Data organizing committee and contributors

BraTS challenge database was prepared with the involvement of following organizers and their institutions: i) Spyridon (Spyros) and Bakas of Center for Biomedical Image Computing and Analytics (CBICA), University of Pennsylvania, USA, ii) Bjoern Menze of Technical University of Munich (TUM), Germany, and iii) Keyvan Farahani of Cancer Imaging Program, National Cancer Institute (NCI), National Institutes of Health, USA, and others.

The database required to prepare BraTS challenge has been contributed by the following institutes: i)The Cancer Imaging Archive (TCIA), Cancer Imaging

Program, NCI, National Institutes of Health (NIH), USA, ii) Center for Biomedical Image Computing and Analytics (CBICA), SBIA, UPenn, PA, USA, iii) University of Alabama at Birmingham, AL, USA, iv) University of Bern, Switzerland, iv) University of Debrecen, Hungarya, and others.

2.5 Conclusions

The tumors can be benign (noncancerous) as well as malignant (cancerous), they have different features and hence can be identified through brain imaging. Different standards of grading the tumors are given by world health organization (WHO), a grade tells the severity of the tumor. Doctors may conclude the type of tumor based on the observations in the brain images and accordingly plan the treatments. The BraTS 2018 database is used for training and evaluation of model performance. In this database, the structural information (subregions) and their labels of brain tumor MR images for segmentation task is discussed. In the next chapter, traditional filters and deep learning models are considered for denoising of brain tumor MR image.

Chapter 3

Denoising of Brain Tumor MR Image

3.1 Introduction

Image denoising technique is used to enhance the quality of images, because while acquiring images they are degraded by different noises. Medical images get corrupted by Gaussian and speckle noises in general. This chapter highlights denoising of brain tumor MR images using the proposed deep learning model (DeepCNN) for different types of noises with known and unknown noise levels. Noisy image is obtained in three ways, by adding Gaussian noise of range 5 to 50, by adding speckle noise of range 5 to 50, and by adding different noises like Gaussian, salt and pepper, Poisson and speckle with a specified noise level of 15. For denoising purpose, various traditional filters like Gaussian, adaptive, bilateral, and guided filters, deep learning models (pretrained DnCNN, proposed deepCNN) are considered. The performance of traditional filters and deep learning models are evaluated in terms of parameters like PSNR, SSIM, MSE, and MAE. This chapter is structured as follows. Section 3.2 presents an overview of various noise types. Denoising of brain tumor MR images using traditional filters is discussed in section 3.3. Advantages of using deep learning, architecture details of pretrained DnCNN and image denoising using this model are described in section 3.4. Section 3.5 focuses on methodologies used for image denoising using proposed DeepCNN model. Section 3.6 discusses the performance metrics to evaluate the models. Section 3.7 deals with experimental results and discussion. Finally, conclusions are given in section 3.8.

3.2 Noise

The MR images are degraded by noise during their acquisition or transmission. Reducing the noise without degrading the quality of an image is called image denoising. Denoising is a part of either preprocessing or in some cases as a component in other process and it is an essential task performed before classification

34

and segmentation of brain tumor MR images. To reinforce the smoothness of the image taken, different algorithms are used for denoising and noises are removed using filtering techniques without affecting the image quality. The noises considered are Gaussian, salt and pepper, speckle and Poisson. Gaussian noise (Zhang K et al., 2017), (Luisier Florian et al., 2011, J Portilla et al., 2003) is evenly distributed over the image and has a normal Gaussian distribution function. Salt and pepper noise has white and black pixels corresponding to the minimum and maximum values. Speckle noise mostly occurs in medical images as a multiplicative noise and has gamma distribution. Poisson noise (Luisier Florian et al., 2011, J Portilla et al., 2003) has Poisson distribution and approximates to Gaussian noise other than very low intensity levels.

3.2.1 Significance of noise

Noise can appear in images from a variety of sources during the acquisition process due to poor resolution of cameras and illumination variations. The noise is undesired in formation that contaminates the image. In image denoising process, information about the type of noise present in the original image plays a significant role. The filter attenuates the noise while preserving details of an image. Noise is present in an image either in additive or multiplicative form. An additive noise (Ponomarenko N, 2005) follows the below Eq. 3.1.

$$w(x,y) = s(x,y) + n(x,y) \tag{3.1}$$

While the multiplicative noise (Aubert G and J F Aujol, 2008) satisfies

$$w(x,y) = s(x,y) \times n(x,y) \tag{3.2}$$

Where, $s(x,y)$ is the original image, $n(x,y)$ denotes the noise introduced to produce the corrupted image $w(x,y)$, and (x,y) represents the pixel location.

3.2.2 Different types of noise in medical images

The different types of noises carried out for denoising purpose discussed in this section are Guassian, salt and pepper, speckle and Poisson.

3.2.2.1 Gaussian noise

Gaussian noise is also known as normal distribution and whose probability density distribution is equal to statistical noise and has mathematical representation of normal distribution. The probability distribution function of normal distribution (Cintra R J et al., 2014) f(x) is given by equation

$$f(x|\mu,\sigma^2) = \frac{1}{\sqrt{2\pi\sigma^2}} e^{\frac{(x-\mu)^2}{2\sigma^2}}$$
(3.3)

Where, μ is the mean or expectation of the distribution, σ is the standard deviation, σ^2 is the variance.

3.2.2.2 Salt and pepper noise

Images with salt and pepper noise generally have bright pixels in dark portion and dark pixels in bright portion. As a result of this noise Black and White dots appear on the images (Sampat M P et al., 2005). This noise arises due to sharp, unexpected changes of image signal, dead pixels, analog to digital converter errors, bit errors in transmission, etc. This kind of noise can be removed by using Dark Frame Subtraction (DFS) and by constructing new data points around dark and bright pixels which is obtained by the median filter or morphological filter (Ning C Y et al., 2009). The mathematical representation of salt & pepper noise is given by

$$P(z)=\begin{cases} p_a & \text{for z=a} \\ p_b & \text{for z=b} \\ 0 & \text{otherwise} \end{cases}$$
(3.4)

If b>a, grey-level b appears as a light dot (salt) in the image. Conversely, a will appear as dark dot (pepper).If either Pa, Pb is zero, the Probability Density Function is called unipolar.

3.2.2.3 Speckle noise

Speckle noise (Marois C et al., 2000) is a phenomenon that conveys all coherent imaging modal quality in which images are produced by interfering echoes of a transmitted waveform that originate from diversity of the studied objects. The speckle noise will appear as bright or dark spots on the image and limits the accuracy of the measurements. This is because the brightness of a pixel is determined not only

36

by properties of the scatterers in the resolution cell, but also by the phase relationships between transmitted and returned signals from those scatterers. Speckle noise is multiplicative in nature, having granular pattern and the traditional filtering cannot remove it easily. Mathematically, speckle noise is expressed by Eq. 3.4.

$$x(i,j) = s(i,j) \times n(i,j) + \eta(i,j) \tag{3.5}$$

Where, $s(i,j)$ is the original image, $n(i,j)$ is the multiplicative noise, $\eta(i,j)$ is the additive noise whose statistics depend on the image and $x(i,j)$ is the corrupted noise image. This kind of noise affects ultrasound and MRI images. The speckle noise limits the efficiency of algorithms in target recognition and texture analysis leading to a grainy appearance in images. Hence, speckle filtering (Szkulmowski M et al., 2012) turns to be a critical preprocessing step for detection or classification. Speckle noise follows gamma distribution as shown below.

$$F(g) = \frac{g^{\alpha-1}}{(\alpha-1)! a^{\alpha}} e^{\frac{-g}{a}} \tag{3.6}$$

Here, $F(g)$ is gamma distribution, g is a random variable (gray level), a is a positive scale parameter, α is a positive shape parameter, and a^{α} is variance.

3.2.2.4 Poisson noise

Poisson noise (Salmon J et al., 2014) is an electronic noise that occurs in an image with the limited number of particles that carry energy, such as electrons in an electronic circuit or photons in photosensitive device. Poisson noise is small enough to give rise to detectable statistical variations in a measurement. Consider a stream of discrete photons emitting from a source and hitting a point to create a visible spot. The physical process that governs the light emission in such a way that photons are emitted from a light source to hit the point many times, such that billions of photons are required to create a visible spot. However, if the source is not able to emit a handful number of photons which hits the point every second, then this noise is caused. This noise is also called as quantum (photon) noise or shot noise.

3.3 Image denoising using traditional filters

Filtering methods are generally preferred for reducing noise in an image. Using traditional filters to reduce various noises are discussed in this section. Denoising forms an important preprocessing step to improve the quality of the image. The denoising filters used in this section are Gaussian, adaptive, bilateral and guided filters.

Adaptive and Gaussian filter denoising methods will result in an edge blurred situation. Bilateral filtering (Zhang Ming et al., 2008, Burger Harold C et al., 2012) is the most intuitive nonlinear smoothing filter which undergoes gradient inversion effect and uses a histogram-based approximation to calculate the weight. As it has computational complexity, Zhang et al. (Zhang Kai et al., 2017) developed an improved bilateral filter based framework capable of efficiently removing universal noise. The bilateral filter takes into account grayscale similarity, spatial information and attains both denoising and edge-preserving. Gradient reverse problem is the drawback in the bilateral filter. The Gaussian filter is unstable when an edge pixel has a few similar pixels around it (Lebrun Marc et al., 2012), (Buades A et al., 2005b).

The image denoising is performed using different filters by adding various types of noises. The application of various filters (Adaptive filter, Gaussian filter, bilateral filter, and guided Filter) for image denoising is presented in Fig. 3.1.

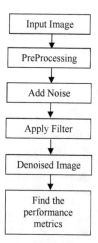

Fig. 3.1 Block diagram of image denoising with various traditional filters.

Figure 3.1 shows the block diagram for the execution of a single brain tumor image. The input image is an RGB image of random size is 705 pixels × 981 pixels × 3 channels. And, it is converted into a grayscale image of size of 256 pixels × 256 pixels × 1 channels channel in preprocessing. Different types of noises like Gaussian noise, salt and pepper noise, speckle noise, and Poisson noise are added to the preprocessed image to form a noisy image. The two frameworks (shown in Fig. 3.3 and 3.4) follow the same procedure to form a noisy image. In the first framework (shown in Fig. 3.1), the noisy image is filtered using different filters such as adaptive filter, Gaussian filter, bilateral filter, and guided filter. From the denoised image, the performance metrics like Peak Signal to Noise Ratio (PSNR in dB), Structural Similarity index of Image (SSIM) Mean Square Error (MSE), and Mean Absolute Error (MAE) are calculated.

Despite most of the methods based on a priori image have high denoising quality, but they are typically suffered from two major drawbacks: i) These methods generally involve a complex optimization problem in the testing stage, making the denoising process time-consuming and hardly achieve high performance without sacrificing computational efficiency. ii) The models are nonconvex and involve several manually chosen parameters, providing some leeway to boost denoising performance. Another nonegligible drawback is that they train a specific model for a certain noise level, and are limited in blind image denoising in addition to this, medical images are inherently complex in structure.

To overcome the limitations of prior-based methods, a discriminative learning method that is DeepCNN model is implemented to get rid of the iterative optimization procedure in the test phase. The image denoising is treated as a plain discriminative learning problem, i.e., separating the noise from a noisy image by feed forward Convolutional Neural Networks (CNN). The reasons of using CNN are three-fold. First, CNN with very deep architecture is effective in increasing the capacity and flexibility to exploit image characteristics. Second, considerable advances have been achieved on regularization and learning methods for training CNN, including Rectifier Linear Unit (ReLU), batch normalization and residual learning. These methods can be adopted to improve denoising performance. Third, CNN is well suited for parallel computation on modern powerful Graphical Processing Unit (GPU) which can be exploited to improve the run time performance.

3.4 Brain tumor MR image denoising using DnCNN

DnCNN is a pretrained Convolutional Neural Network (CNN) (Jain Viren et al., 2009, Xiao Ping Zhang, 2001) for image regression problem. It contains an input layer, convolutional layers, batch normalization layer, rectifier linear unit layer, max pooling layer, dense or fully connect layer, and finally regression layer. Usually, it is also called as a multilayer neural network. The structural design of a CNN (K Simonyan and A Zisserman, 2015, S Gu et al., 2014, A Buades et al., 2005a) is planned to get the benefit of the 2D arrangement of an input image. This is attained with local networks and weights monitored by a certain method of pooling (Mao Xiaojiao et al., 2016) which effects translation invariant features. CNN models (DnCNN) for brain tumor MR image denoising is chosen because of three reasons. First, a very deep architecture of the CNN increases the flexibility and capacity for exploiting the image characteristics. Second, the CNN speeds up the training process and improves the performance of denoising due to sparsity (W Dong et at., 2015), weight sharing, batch normalization, and ReLU. Third, parallel computing capabilities of CNN on modern powerful GPU is used to improve the run-time performance.

3.4.1 Architecture of pretrained DnCNN model

There are many pretrained convolutional neural networks for regression problems and image classification (Zhang Y D et al., 2011, Wang Q et al., 2018). The DnCNN (Zhang Kai et al., 2017, K Simonyan et al., 2015) is a 20 convolutional layers depth pretrained model for performing image denoising task. It contains totally 59 layers including one input layer, 20 convolutional layers, 19 ReLU layers, 18 batch normalization layers, and one regression output layer. The architecture of DnCNN model is shown in Fig. 3.2.

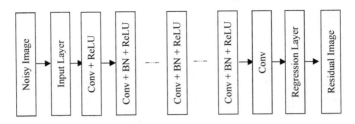

Fig. 3.2 Architecture of DnCNN model.

In this architecture model, the pooling layers are avoided. The model has three different types of layers as shown in Fig. 3.2. The Conv+ReLU is the first convolutional layer, which is used after the input layer (patch size, patch size, channels). In this architecture, the convolutional layer is followed by activation layer, ReLU. All convolutional layers use filters of size 3 pixels × 3 pixels × channels (of size 64 filters) to generate 64 feature maps. Here, channels = 1 for gray image and 3 for RGB image. The Conv+BN+ReLU is a combination of three layers, convolutional, batch normalization, and ReLU layer. In the proposed model, this combination is repeated 18 times between first Conv+ReLU layer and last convolutional layer, Conv20. Sixty four filters of size 3 × 3 × 64 are used and batch normalization layer is added between Convolutional layer and ReLU layer. The Conv is the last convolutional layer, number of filters of size 3 × 3 × 64 are utilized to reproduce the output. The final layer in the model is the regression layer to calculate the mean squares error.

3.4.2 Image denoising using DnCNN

The second framework details the application of DnCNN for image denoising. In the second framework (Fig. 3.3), one of the pretrained convolutional neural network (DnCNN) is considered for denoising. The DnCNN is well trained on millions of natural images database, ImageNet. Load well optimised weights of DnCNN as network or model, then pass the DnCNN network and a noisy 2D image to reduce the noise. Then the performance metrics are calculated from the denoised image. The below Fig. 3.3 shows the workflow to denoise an image using the pretrained DnCNN network.

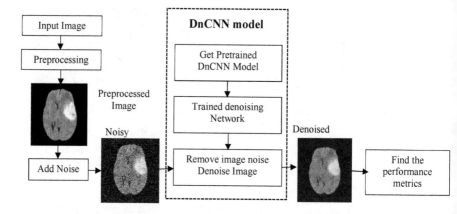

Fig. 3.3 Framework of image denoising with pretrained convolutional neural networks (DnCNNs).

The simplest and fastest solution is to use the built-in pretrained denoising neural network, called DnCNN and it is directly considered for noise removal. However, the pretrained network does not offer much flexibility in the case of recognized types of noises because the network or model is not trained with BraTS dataset here.

The pretrained DnCNN network is used to remove Gaussian noise without the challenge of training a network. Removing noise with the pretrained network has the following limitations:

- Noise removal works only with 2D single channel images. If there are multiple color channels or 3D images, noise can be removed by treating each channel or plane separately.
- The network recognizes only Gaussian noise, with a limited range of standard deviation.

To overcome limitations of this frame work, to get more flexibility and improve the denoising performance, the network has to be trained using predefined layers and customize denoising neural network.

3.5 Brain tumor MR image denoising using proposed DeepCNN Model

In this section, the proposed DL model (DeepCNN) and image denoising using proposed model are discussed.

3.5.1 Architecture of proposed deep learning model (DeepCNN)

Architecture of proposed DeepCNN model is same as DnCNN architecture. But it is a 17 convolutional layers depth model and has 50 layers including one input layer, 17 convolutional layers, 16 ReLU layers, 15 batch normalization layers, and one regression output layer. The input layer used for DnCNN is an image of patch size 50×50, whereas patch size 61×61 can be used as the input layer image size in DeepCNN. Moreover, it offers favorable results when extended to numerous traditional images denoising tasks.

One important issue of the model architecture is to fix proper depth for better performance and efficiency. The depth of the model is dependent on effective patch size and noise level in the image. Usually high noise level image denoising task requires large effective patch size. Here the proposed DeepCNN model learns to estimate the residual image. The residual image contains information about the image distortion. The denoised image is obtained by subtracting residual image from original image.

Due to batch normalization, ReLU, and 17 convolutional layers, the training process gets speeded up, boost the denoising performance and over fitting problem is also avoided by doing augmentation of the datasets. So the proposed DeepCNN model gives better performance in achieving denoising than other methods.

3.5.2 Image denoising using proposed DeepCNN

A model is trained to detect a larger range of Gaussian noise standard deviations from grayscale images, starting with predefined layers. To train a denoising model using predefined layers, the steps followed are,

- Create an image data store that stores original images.

- Create a denoising image data store that generates noisy training data from the original images in the image data store. Here noise level, patch size, and channel format are specified, so that the size of the training data matches the input size of the network.
- Get the predefined DnCNN layers as network or model.
- Define training options to train the model. The training options are adam optimizer, Maximum Epochs 30, Initial learn rate 0.0001, and Mini batch size 16.
- Train the network specifying the denoising image data store as the data source.

For each iteration of training, the denoising image data store generates one mini-batch of training data by randomly cropping original images from the image data store, then adding randomly generated zero-mean Gaussian white noise to each image patch. The standard deviation of the added noise is unique for each image patch, and has a value within the range specified by the noise level of the denoising image data store. After the network has trained, pass the network and a noisy image to denoise image. The training and denoising workflow are shown in Fig. 3.4.

BraTS 2018 database is considered to prepare the image data store size of 400 images and used for training the DeepCNN model. Patches (D Zoran and Y Weiss, 2011) are extracted with an effective patch size of 61 at the rate of 64 patches per image. Denoising image data store is prepared by using these patches with Gaussian noise of noise level range from 5 to 50. DeepCNN model is then trained to this dataset to perform the denoising task. The noisy image is applied to the DeepCNN model to reduce the noise in the image. The performance metrics are calculated from the denoised image.

This work is carried out for Gaussian noise with noise level range from 5 to 50. The results of proposed DeepCNN model is compared with pretrained DnCNN and the filters stated above (bilateral filter, adaptive filter, Gaussian filter, and guided filter). The proposed DeepCNN method has achieved superior PSNR, SSIM, MSE, and MAE in terms of performance metrics.

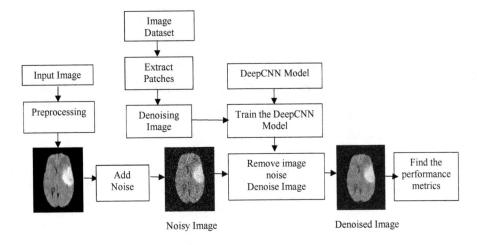

Noisy Image   Denoised Image

Fig. 3.4 Framework of image denoising with proposed DeepCNN.

3.6 Performance evaluation metrics

The performance of discussed methods is measured in terms of PSNR in dB, SSIM, MSE, and MAE.

PSNR: PSNR of an image is the noise immunity indicated by peak signal to noise ratio. High PSNR value indicates less interference in the MRI brain image due to noise. Generally, PSNR can be expressed by the following expression.

$$PSNR = 10 \log_{10}\left(\frac{MAX_i^2}{MSE}\right) = 20 \log_{10}\left(\frac{MAX_i}{\sqrt{MSE}}\right) \qquad (3.7)$$

Where max_i denotes the highest pixel value in the input brain tumor MR image and MSE denotes the mean square error.

Typical values for the PSNR in noisy image and original image are between 30 and 50 dB, provided the bit depth is 8 bits, where higher is better. For 16-bit data typical values for the PSNR are between 60 and 80 dB.

SSIM: It is a technique for guessing the perceived feature of digital TV and photographic pictures, as well as other types of digital images and videos. It is nearer to the human insight that it reflects the resemblance in structural information of image pairs.

45

It calculates a P test image with respect to a Q reference image to measure their visual similarity. P and Q are the images to be compared $p = \{p_i | i=1,2,...N\}$ and $q = \{q_i | i=1,2,...N\}$ are of local square pairs of P and Q respectively. At same spatial location, p and q are positioned in the images. The terms used in SSIM are μ_p average pixel values, constant C, standard deviations of pixel (SD), σ_p and σ_q at patches p and q and cross-correlation (covariance) σ_{pq} of p and q.

$$l(p,q) = \left(2\mu_p\mu_q + C1\right)/\left(\mu_p^2 + \mu_q^2 + C1\right) \tag{3.8}$$

$$c(p,q) = \left(2\sigma_p\sigma_q + C2\right)/\left(\sigma_p^2 + \sigma_q^2 + C2\right) \tag{3.9}$$

$$r(p,q) = \left(\sigma_{pq} + C3\right)/\left(\sigma_p\sigma_q + C3\right) \tag{3.10}$$

Where, the constants C1, C2, and C3 are considered to be stable. When $(\mu_p^2 + \mu_q^2)$, $(\sigma_p^2 + \sigma_q^2)$ or $\sigma_p\sigma_q$ is set to zero. The $l(p,q)$ index stands for the luminance differences, $c(p,q)$ stands for contrast differences, and $r(p,q)$ stands for the structural variations between x and y.

Now the SSIM index is stated as

$$SSIM(p,q) = [l(p,q)]^\alpha \cdot [c(p,q)]^\beta \cdot [r(p,q)]^\gamma \tag{3.11}$$

Where, α, β, and γ are the parameters to describe the comparative significance of each component and SSIM(p,q) ranges from 0 (fully diverse) to 1 (identical patches).

The SSIM values range from 0 to 1, if SSIM is 1 means that the reconstructed image structurally closed to original one. Generally SSIM values 0.97, 0.98, 0.99 for good quality reconstruction techniques.

MSE: Mean Squared Error is the quality measurement of the image. It can be expressed as the cumulative squared error value between the input images R (a, b) and the segmented image input images.

$$MSE = \frac{1}{mn}\sum_{a=0}^{m-1}\sum_{b=0}^{n-1}\left[R(a,b) - D(a,b)\right]^2 \tag{3.12}$$

Where 'm' is the number of rows and 'n' is the number of columns in the input image. PSNR value is inversely proportional to the MSE value. An image should have high PSNR and low MSE for best quality.

MAE: Mean Absolute Error is the quality measurement of the image. It can be expressed as the cumulative absolute error value between the input images R (a, b) and the segmented image D (a, b).

$$MAE = \frac{1}{mn} \sum_{a=0}^{m-1} \sum_{b=0}^{n-1} |R(a,b)-D(a,b)| \qquad (3.13)$$

Where, 'm' is the number of rows and 'n' is the number of columns in the input image. PSNR value is inversely proportional to the MAE value.

The mean-absolute error (MAE), the mean-square error (MSE), and peak signal-to-noise ratio (PSNR) are used to compare image denoise quality. The MSE represents the cumulative squared error between the denoised and the original image, whereas MAE represents the absolute error between the denoised and the original image. The lower the value of MSE, the lower the error. The PSNR computes the peak signal-to-noise ratio, in decibels, between two images. This ratio is used as a quality measurement between the original and a denoised image. The higher the PSNR, the better the quality of the denoised, or reconstructed image.

3.7 Experimental results and discussions

In this section, images considered for denoising task are corrupted in three ways. Firstly, image is corrupted by adding Gaussian noise with wide range of noise level from 5 to 50. Second, image is corrupted by adding speckle noise with wide range of noise level from 5 to 50. Third, image is corrupted by adding different noises like Gaussian, salt and pepper, Poisson, and speckle noise with a specified noise level of 15. The experimental results of all these cases are obtained using traditional filters, DnCNN, and proposed DeepCNN model and discussed in sections 3.3, 3.4, and 3.5 respectively. The entire denoising work is executed on the system with specifications of core i5, 7th generation Intel processor with 8GB RAM and GPU of 4GB NVIDIA graphic card.

Consider the first case where the image is corrupted by adding Gaussian noise with wide range of noise level from 5 to 50.

47

Sl.No.	Denoising images
1	Noise level $\sigma = 5$

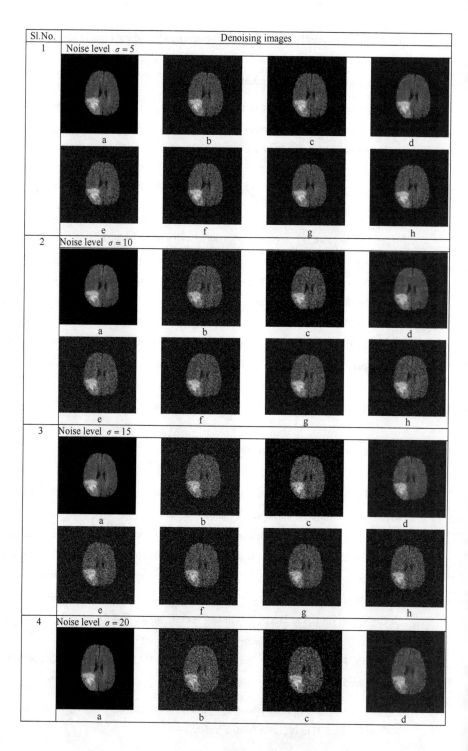

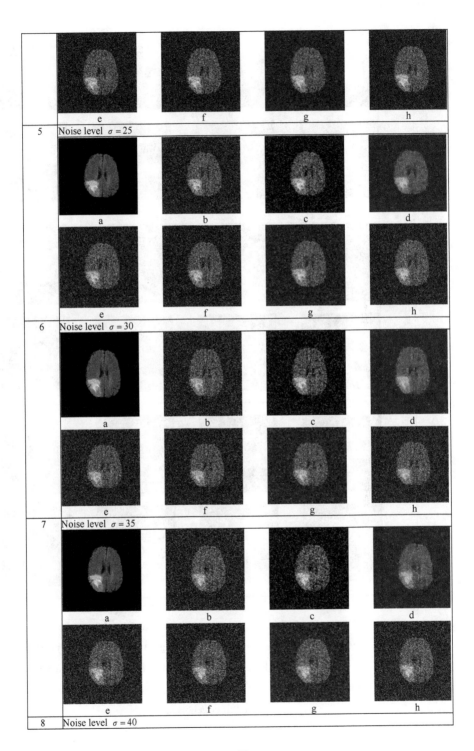

	e	f	g	h
5	Noise level $\sigma = 25$			
	a	b	c	d
	e	f	g	h
6	Noise level $\sigma = 30$			
	a	b	c	d
	e	f	g	h
7	Noise level $\sigma = 35$			
	a	b	c	d
	e	f	g	h
8	Noise level $\sigma = 40$			

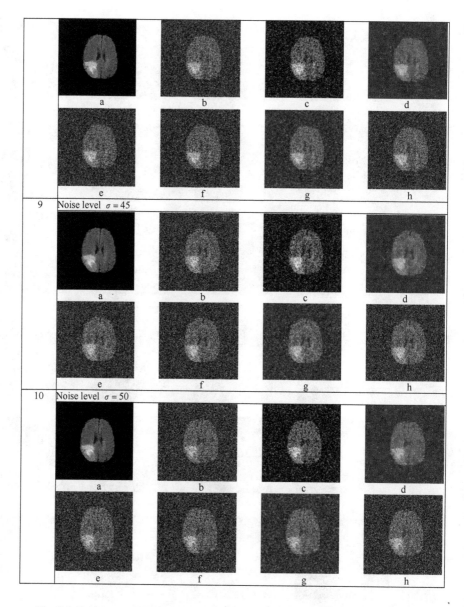

Fig. 3.5 Brain tumor MR image denoising with various Gaussian noise level range from 5 to 50 (from Sl.No. 1 to 10). a) Original images b) Noisy images c) Pretrained DnCNN denoised images d) Proposed DeepCNN denoised images e) Gaussian filter denoised images f) Bilateral filter denoised images g) Adaptive filter denoised images h) Guided filter denoised images.

Figure 3.5 shows the noise removal of brain tumor MR images, when the image is corrupted by Gaussian noise with noise level range of 5 to 50. Original images and noisy images are shown in Fig. 3.5 a and b, respectively, from Sl.No. 1 to 10. Here, the denoised images obtained by various models and filters like pretrained DnCNN model, proposed DeepCNN model, Gaussian filter, bilateral filter, adaptive filter, and guided filter are shown in Fig. 3.5 c to h, respectively, from Sl.No. 1 to 10. Among all filters and pretrained DnCNN method, the proposed DeepCNN gives clear denoised image visually.

Table 3.1 Performance evaluation metrics of proposed DeepCNN, pretrained DnCNN, Gaussian, adaptive, bilateral, and guided filters with Gaussian noise from noise level 5 to 50.

Sl.No	Noise Level	Method	PSNR (dB)	SSIM	MSE	MAE
1	σ = 5	DeepCNN	**28.9274**	**0.2385**	**83.242**	**7.9241**
		DnCNN	25.3215	0.1931	192.5861	12.122
		Gaussian Filter	22.0212	0.1021	408.2814	13.1201
		Adaptive Filter	23.5891	0.121	284.5587	12.9042
		Guided Filter	22.5777	0.0948	359.1772	13.3766
		Bilateral Filter	19.376	0.0702	750.7282	14.0564
2	σ = 10	DeepCNN	**25.3826**	**0.1978**	**192.6814**	**12.112**
		DnCNN	22.4189	0.1631	375.0291	16.8145
		Gaussian Filter	19.0666	0.0711	806.1604	18.3615
		Adaptive Filter	20.6993	0.0842	553.5446	18.0257
		Guided Filter	18.7139	0.0566	874.3521	18.9955
		Bilateral Filter	16.4364	0.0466	1.48E+03	19.6528
3	σ = 15	DeepCNN	**22.39**	**0.1587**	**375.0389**	**16.7951**
		DnCNN	20.6479	0.1391	559.042	20.6937
		Gaussian Filter	17.3626	0.0581	1.19E+03	22.6497
		Adaptive Filter	19.0365	0.0698	811.7672	22.2023
		Guided Filter	16.5214	0.0432	1.45E+03	23.5897
		Bilateral Filter	14.7473	0.0372	2.18E+03	24.2206
4	σ = 20	DeepCNN	**20.6564**	**0.1412**	**559.042**	**20.6937**
		DnCNN	19.439	0.119	738.3465	23.6042
		Gaussian Filter	16.2135	0.0487	1.56E+03	25.9013
		Adaptive Filter	17.9776	0.0605	1.04E+03	25.2583
		Guided Filter	15.1004	0.0343	2.01E+03	27.0262
		Bilateral Filter	13.6152	0.03	2.83E+03	27.6357
5	σ = 25	DeepCNN	**19.448**	**0.125**	**738.3745**	**23.7842**
		DnCNN	18.5059	0.1099	911.2204	26.3927
		Gaussian Filter	15.3035	0.0445	1.92E+03	28.8271
		Adaptive Filter	17.1165	0.0554	1.26E+03	28.0908

		Guided Filter	14.0023	0.0305	2.59E+03	30.1588
		Bilateral Filter	12.7315	0.0272	3.47E+03	30.7473
6	σ = 30	DeepCNN	**18.506**	**0.1169**	**917.2244**	**26.4804**
		DnCNN	17.6692	0.1029	1.10E+03	29.3711
		Gaussian Filter	14.5256	0.0394	2.29E+03	31.774
		Adaptive Filter	16.3852	0.051	1.49E+03	30.8846
		Guided Filter	13.0924	0.0264	3.19E+03	33.2674
		Bilateral Filter	11.9823	0.0237	4.12E+03	33.8356
7	σ = 35	DeepCNN	**17.6741**	**0.1031**	**1.11E+03**	**29.2791**
		DnCNN	16.8921	0.0968	1.20E+03	31.5921
		Gaussian Filter	13.8871	0.0358	2.66E+03	34.278
		Adaptive Filter	15.8055	0.049	1.71E+03	33.1749
		Guided Filter	12.3398	0.0232	3.79E+03	35.9218
		Bilateral Filter	11.3528	0.021	4.76E+03	36.484
8	σ = 40	DeepCNN	**16.9834**	**0.0979**	**1.30E+03**	**31.6065**
		DnCNN	16.4132	0.0924	1.48E+03	33.4921
		Gaussian Filter	13.466	0.0346	2.93E+03	36.2189
		Adaptive Filter	15.4271	0.0489	1.86E+03	34.9752
		Guided Filter	11.864	0.022	4.23E+03	37.9388
		Bilateral Filter	10.9496	0.0199	5.23E+03	38.4968
9	σ = 45	DeepCNN	**16.5299**	**0.0934**	**1.45E+03**	**33.4439**
		DnCNN	15.9954	0.0861	1.61E+03	35.6172
		Gaussian Filter	12.9662	0.0319	3.28E+03	38.4249
		Adaptive Filter	14.9504	0.0468	2.08E+03	37.0855
		Guided Filter	11.3173	0.0203	4.80E+03	40.214
		Bilateral Filter	10.4811	0.0184	5.82E+03	40.7678
10	σ = 50	DeepCNN	**15.9539**	**0.0851**	**1.65E+03**	**35.6019**
		DnCNN	15.5281	0.0805	1.82E+03	37.3686
		Gaussian Filter	12.5788	0.0307	3.59E+03	40.2788
		Adaptive Filter	14.5842	0.046	2.26E+03	38.8006
		Guided Filter	10.8701	0.0191	5.32E+03	42.1916
		Bilateral Filter	10.0962	0.0174	6.36E+03	42.7376

Table 3.1 presents the performance metrics of proposed DeepCNN, DnCNN methods, and other filtering methods with varying levels of Gaussian noise for denoising. It is clear that with increasing noise content the PSNR and SSIM values decrease. For one instant noise level sigma equal to 20, the de noising performance metrics of DeepCNN like PSNR in dB, SSIM, MSE, and MAE are 20.6564, 0.1412, 559.042, and 20.6937 respectively. From table 1 the proposed DeepCNN model shows superior performance when compared with DnCNN and all filtering methods with unknown noise level of Gaussian noise. Hence DeepCNN seems to be the better

suitable method for reducing noise when the image is corrupted by the known or unknown level of Gaussian noise.

Figure 3.6 shows the variation of PSNR with different noise level ranging from 5 to 50 for different filters (Gaussian Filter (GAF), Adaptive Filter (AF), Guided Filter (GUF), Bilateral Filter (BF)), and models (pretrained DnCNN and proposed DeepCNN). The proposed DeepCNN gives a highest PSNR and decreases with increasing noise level when compared with other filters and models by adding Gaussian noise.

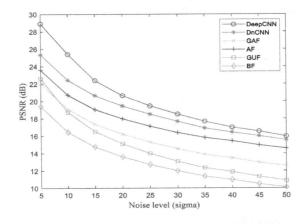

Fig. 3.6 Plot of PSNR values in dB versus Gaussian noise level for various denoising methods.

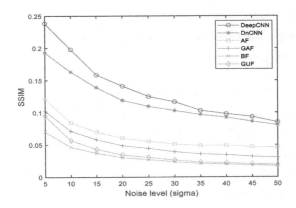

Fig. 3.7 Plot of SSIM values versus Gaussian noise level for various denoising methods.

Figure 3.7 shows the variation of SSIM with different noise level ranging from 5 to 50 for different filters (Gaussian Filter (GAF), Bilateral Filter (BF), Adaptive Filter (AF), Guided Filter (GUF)), and models (pretrained DnCNN and proposed DeepCNN). The proposed DeepCNN gives a better SSIM of 0.2385 and decreases with increasing noise level when compared with other filters and models by adding Gaussian noise.

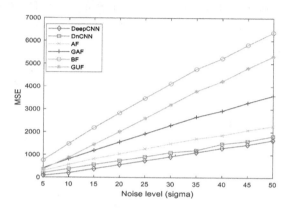

Fig. 3.8 Plot of MSE values versus Gaussian noise level for various denoising methods.

Figure 3.8 shows the variation of MSE with different noise level ranging from 5 to 50 for different filters (Gaussian Filter (GAF), Bilateral Filter (BF), Adaptive Filter (AF), Guided Filter (GUF)), and models (pretrained DnCNN and proposed DeepCNN). The proposed DeepCNN gives a minimum MSE value and increases with increasing noise level when compared with other filters and models by adding Gaussian noise.

Figure 3.9 shows the variation of MAE with different noise level sigma ranging from 5 to 50 for different filters (Gaussian Filter (GAF), Bilateral Filter (BF), Adaptive Filter (AF), Guided Filter (GUF)), and models (pretrained DnCNN and proposed DeepCNN). The proposed DeepCNN gives a minimum MAE value and increases with increasing noise level when compared with other filters and models by adding Gaussian noise.

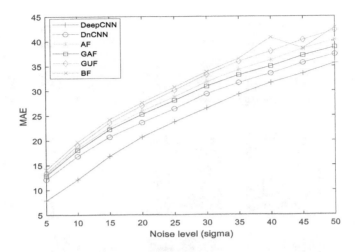

Fig. 3.9 Plot of MAE values versus Gaussian noise level for various denoising
methods.

Consider the second case where the image is corrupted by adding speckle
noise with a wide range of noise level from 5 to 50.

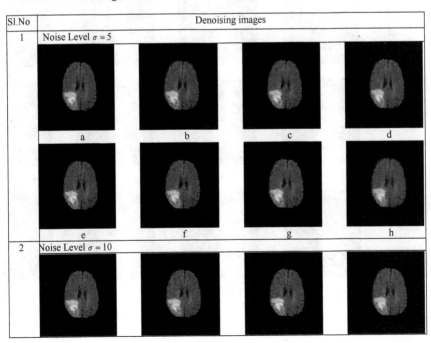

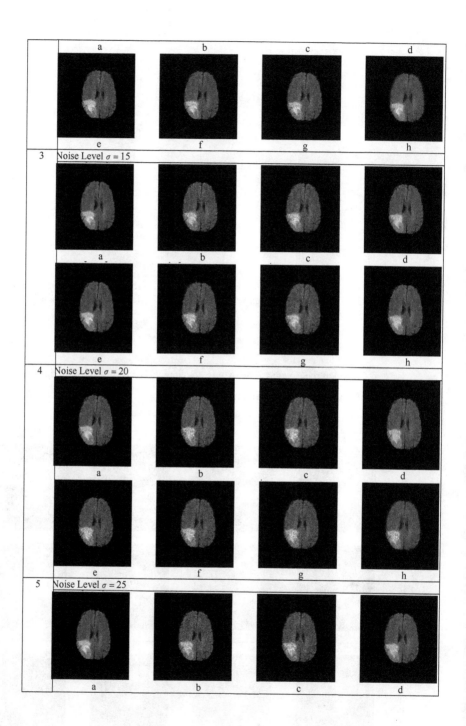

| | a | b | c | d |
| | e | f | g | h |

3 | Noise Level $\sigma = 15$

| | a | b | c | d |
| | e | f | g | h |

4 | Noise Level $\sigma = 20$

| | a | b | c | d |
| | e | f | g | h |

5 | Noise Level $\sigma = 25$

| | a | b | c | d |

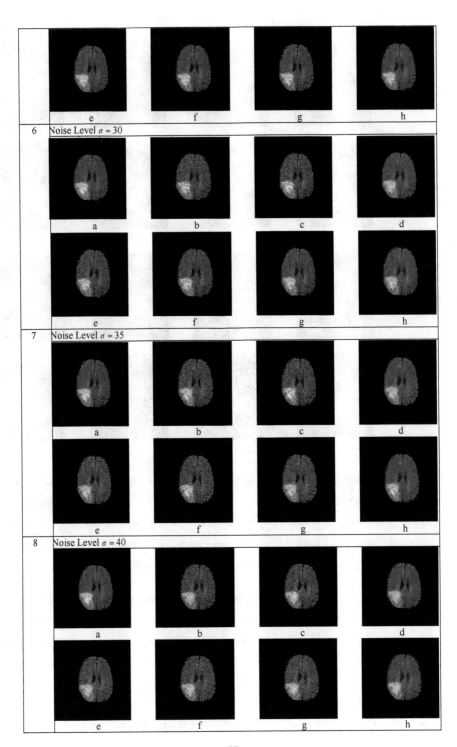

| e | f | g | h |

6 | Noise Level $\sigma = 30$

| a | b | c | d |

| e | f | g | h |

7 | Noise Level $\sigma = 35$

| a | b | c | d |

| e | f | g | h |

8 | Noise Level $\sigma = 40$

| a | b | c | d |

| e | f | g | h |

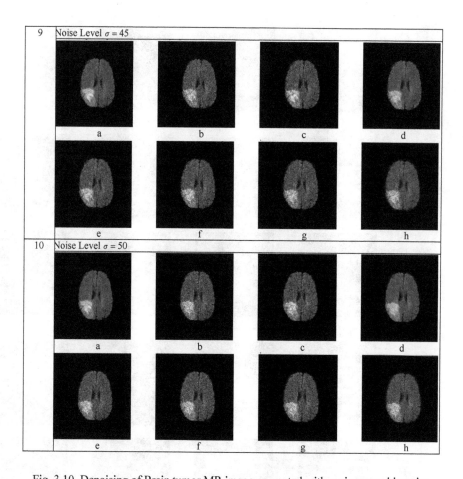

Fig. 3.10 Denoising of Brain tumor MR image corrupted with various speckle noise
level range from 5 to 50 (from Sl.No. 1 to 10). a) Original images b) Noisy images
c) Denoised images using pretrained DnCNN d) Proposed DeepCNN denoised
images e) Gaussian filter denoised images f) Bilateral filter denoised images
g) Adaptive filter denoised images h) Guided filter denoised images.

Figure 3.10 shows the noise removal of brain tumor MR images, where the
image is corrupted by speckle noise with noise level range from 5 to 50. Original
images and noisy images are shown in Fig. 3.10 a and b, respectively, from Sl.No. 1
to 10 starting from noise level of 5 and in increment of 5. Here, the denoised images
obtained by various models and filters like pretrained DnCNN model, proposed
DeepCNN model, Gaussian filter, bilateral filter, adaptive filter, and guided filter are
shown in Fig. 3.10 c to h, respectively, from Sl.No. 1 to 10. Among all the four filters

and pretrained DnCNN model, the proposed DeepCNN gives clear denoised image visually.

Table 3.2   Performance evaluation metrics of proposed DeepCNN, pretrained DnCNN, Gaussian, adaptive, bilateral, and guided filters with speckle noise from various noise level 5 to 50.

Sl.No.	Noise Level	Method	PSNR (dB)	SSIM	MSE	MAE
1	σ = 5	DnCNN	36.625	0.9547	14.1444	0.556
		DeepCNN	**39.4316**	**0.9705**	**7.4118**	**0.5178**
		Gaussian Filter	36.6841	0.9544	13.953	0.6766
		Bilateral Filter	37.1663	0.9667	12.4868	0.5652
		Adaptive Filter	35.5314	0.9557	18.1945	0.7181
		Guided Filter	35.7749	0.9454	17.2023	0.7506
2	σ = 10	DnCNN	34.4705	0.9368	23.2292	0.7523
		DeepCNN	**37.6716**	**0.9611**	**11.1152**	**0.6611**
		Gaussian Filter	33.839	0.9298	26.8644	0.9738
		Bilateral Filter	33.4552	0.9405	29.3469	0.9022
		Adaptive Filter	32.2648	0.9258	38.6014	1.0963
		Guided Filter	33.8835	0.9316	26.5905	0.9357
3	σ = 15	DnCNN	33.2209	0.9256	30.9734	0.7869
		DeepCNN	**36.5237**	**0.9568**	**14.4782**	**0.6599**
		Gaussian Filter	32.2283	0.9154	38.9267	1.0902
		Bilateral Filter	31.3022	0.9189	48.1795	1.1019
		Adaptive Filter	30.4614	0.9064	58.4714	1.2945
		Guided Filter	32.2292	0.916	38.9189	1.046
4	σ = 20	DnCNN	32.1186	0.9131	39.9225	0.9878
		DeepCNN	**35.7782**	**0.9512**	**17.1894**	**0.7507**
		Gaussian Filter	31.0491	0.9038	51.071	1.2896
		Bilateral Filter	29.5764	0.9	71.6874	1.418
		Adaptive Filter	29.1363	0.892	79.3326	1.5609
		Guided Filter	30.8004	0.9001	54.08	1.2768
5	σ = 25	DnCNN	31.3743	0.9066	47.386	0.9893
		DeepCNN	**35.2188**	**0.9476**	**19.5525**	**0.7425**
		Gaussian Filter	30.1705	0.8946	62.5216	1.3831
		Bilateral Filter	28.3862	0.8861	94.2891	1.6035
		Adaptive Filter	28.2123	0.8815	98.1417	1.6957
		Guided Filter	29.725	0.8866	69.2762	1.413
6	σ = 30	DnCNN	30.7113	0.8992	55.2009	1.1387
		DeepCNN	**34.5764**	**0.9436**	**22.6695**	**0.8119**
		Gaussian Filter	29.4205	0.8871	74.3079	1.5296
		Bilateral Filter	27.4065	0.8756	118.1493	1.8488
		Adaptive Filter	27.4384	0.8735	117.2847	1.8869
		Guided Filter	28.7844	0.8761	86.028	1.6051

		DnCNN	29.916	0.8905	66.2944	1.3151
		DeepCNN	**34.1029**	**0.9392**	**25.2807**	**0.882**
7	σ = 35	Gaussian Filter	28.7188	0.8798	87.3382	1.692
		Bilateral Filter	26.4438	0.8662	147.4692	2.1141
		Adaptive Filter	26.6996	0.8663	139.0353	2.0775
		Guided Filter	27.8287	0.8666	107.2032	1.817
		DnCNN	29.259	0.8872	77.1217	1.3396
		DeepCNN	**33.3072**	**0.9344**	**30.3642**	**0.9056**
8	σ = 40	Gaussian Filter	28.0696	0.8755	101.4191	1.7761
		Bilateral Filter	25.6944	0.8602	175.2434	2.2819
		Adaptive Filter	26.085	0.8613	160.1701	2.1928
		Guided Filter	27.047	0.86	128.3441	1.9531
		DnCNN	29.1481	0.8839	79.1169	1.4303
		DeepCNN	**33.2201**	**0.9336**	**30.9789**	**0.9426**
9	σ = 45	Gaussian Filter	27.7547	0.8717	109.0463	1.879
		Bilateral Filter	25.2911	0.8552	192.2946	2.4472
		Adaptive Filter	25.7684	0.857	172.2814	2.322
		Guided Filter	26.6627	0.8545	140.2188	2.0957
		DnCNN	28.7149	0.8776	87.4166	1.5094
		DeepCNN	**33.041**	**0.9299**	**32.2837**	**0.9595**
10	σ = 50	Gaussian Filter	27.3399	0.866	119.9757	1.9746
		Bilateral Filter	24.7914	0.8494	215.7425	2.6143
		Adaptive Filter	25.3453	0.8497	189.9116	2.4458
		Guided Filter	26.1211	0.8483	158.8421	2.2461

Table 3.2 presents the performance metrics obtained by the proposed DeepCNN, pretrained DnCNN model, and other filtering methods along with the varying noise levels for denoising task. It is clear that with decreasing noise content the PSNR and SSIM values increases. For one instant noise level equal to 10, the denoising performance metrics of proposed DeepCNN like PSNR in dB, SSIM, MSE, and MAE are 39.4316, 0.9705, 7.4118, and 0.5178 respectively. From table 3.2, it is evident that the proposed DeepCNN model shows superior performance when compared with pretrained DnCNN and all filtering methods with unknown noise level of speckle noise. It can be concluded that the proposed DeepCNN is a better suitable method for reducing noise when the image is corrupted by the unknown noise level of speckle noise than Gaussian noise.

Figure 3.11 shows the variation of PSNR with different noise level ranging from 5 to 50 for different filters (Gaussian Filter (GAF), Bilateral Filter (BF), Adaptive Filter (AF), Guided Filter (GUF)), and models (pretrained DnCNN and proposed DeepCNN). It can be observed from Fig. 3.11 that the proposed DeepCNN gives a highest PSNR in dB of 39.4316 and decreases with increasing noise level when compared with other filters and models for speckle noise addition.

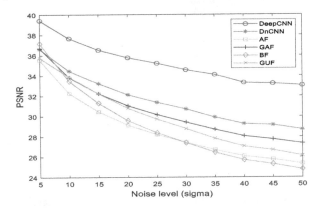

Fig. 3.11 Plot of PSNR values versus speckle noise level for various denoising methods.

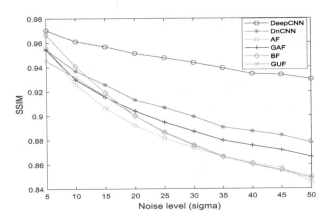

Fig. 3.12 Plot of SSIM values versus speckle noise level for various denoising methods.

Figure 3.12 shows the variation of SSIM with different noise level ranging from 5 to 50 for different filters (Gaussian Filter (GAF), Bilateral Filter (BF), Adaptive Filter (AF), Guided Filter (GUF)), and models (pretrained DnCNN and proposed DeepCNN). It can be observed from Fig. 3.12 that the proposed DeepCNN gives a better SSIM of 0.9705 and decreases with increasing noise level when compared with other filters and models for speckle noise addition.

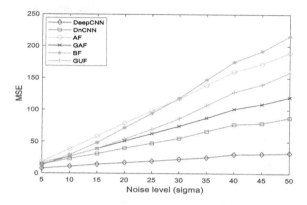

Fig. 3.13 Plot of MSE values versus speckle noise level for various denoising methods

Figure 3.13 shows the variation of MSE with different noise level ranging from 5 to 50 for different filters (Gaussian Filter (GAF), Bilateral Filter (BF), Adaptive Filter (AF), Guided Filter (GUF)), and models (pretrained DnCNN and proposed DeepCNN). It can be observed from the above figure that the proposed DeepCNN gives a minimum MSE value of 7.4118 and increases with increasing noise level when compared with other filters and models for speckle noise addition.

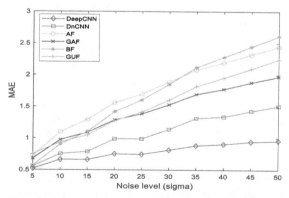

Fig. 3.14 Plot of MAE values versus speckle noise level for various denoising methods.

Figure 3.14 shows the variation of MAE with different noise level sigma ranging from 5 to 50 for different filters (Gaussian Filter (GAF), Bilateral Filter (BF),

Adaptive Filter (AF), Guided Filter (GUF)), and models (pretrained DnCNN and proposed DeepCNN). It can be observed from the above figure that the proposed DeepCNN gives a minimum MAE value of 0.5178 and increases with increasing sigma value when compared with other filters and models for speckle noise addition.

Consider the third case, where image is corrupted by adding different noises with specified noise level of 15. In this case the noisy image is formed by adding different kind of noises like Gaussian noise, salt and pepper noise, Poisson noise, and speckle noise separately with specified noise level of 15.

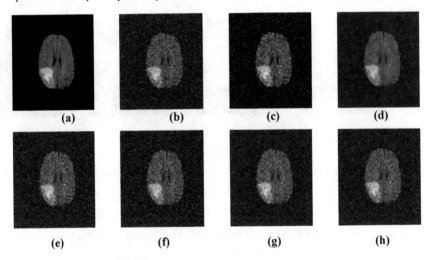

Fig. 3.15 Brain tumor MR image denoising with Gaussian noise of level 15.
a) Original image b) Noisy image c) Pretrained DnCNN denoised images
d) Proposed DeepCNN denoised images e) Gaussian filter denoised images
f) Bilateral filter denoised images g) Adaptive filter denoised images
h) Guided filter denoised images.

Figure 3.15 shows the noise removal of brain tumor MR images, when the image is corrupted by known Gaussian noise of level 15. Original images and noisy images are shown in Fig. 3.15 a and b, respectively. Here, the denoised images obtained by various models and filters like pretrained DnCNN model, proposed DeepCNN model, Gaussian filter, bilateral filter, adaptive filter, and guided filter are shown in Fig. 3.15 c to h respectively. Among all filters and pertained DnCNN, the proposed DeepCNN provides better PSNR and SSIM in terms of performance. It is concluded that the proposed DeepCNN is the best suitable method for reducing noise when the image is corrupted by Gaussian noise with known noise level.

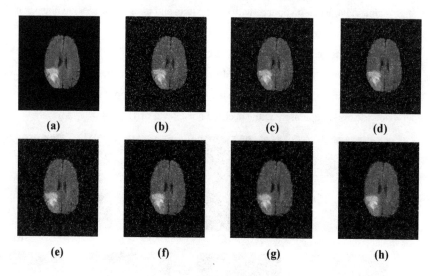

(a)   (b)   (c)   (d)

(e)   (f)   (g)   (h)

Fig. 3.16 Brain tumor MR image denoising with salt and pepper noise level 15.
a) Original image b) Noisy image c) Pretrained DnCNN denoised images
d) Proposed DeepCNN denoised images e) Gaussian filter denoised images
f) Bilateral filter denoised images g) Adaptive filter denoised images
h) Guided filter denoised images.

Figure 3.16 shows the noise removal of brain tumor MR images, when the image is corrupted by known salt and pepper noise level 15. Original images and noisy images are shown in Fig. 3.16 a and b, respectively. Here, the denoised images obtained by various models and filters like pretrained DnCNN model, proposed DeepCNN model, Gaussian filter, bilateral filter, adaptive filter, and guided filter are shown in Fig. 3.16 c to h respectively. Among all filters and pretrained DnCNN, the proposed DeepCNN provides better PSNR and SSIM in terms of performance up to salt and pepper noise level 15 only. The conclusion from Fig. 3.16 is that the proposed DeepCNN is not suitable for reducing noise when the image is corrupted by salt and pepper noise with more than noise level 15.

Figure 3.17 shows the noise removal of brain tumor MR images, when the image is corrupted by known Poisson noise level of 15. Original images and noisy images are shown in Fig. 3.17 a and b, respectively. Here, the denoised images obtained by various models and filters like pretrained DnCNN model, proposed DeepCNN model, Gaussian filter, bilateral filter, adaptive filter, and guided filter are shown in Fig. 3.17 c to h respectively. Among all filters and pertained DnCNN, the proposed DeepCNN provides better PSNR and SSIM in terms of performance.

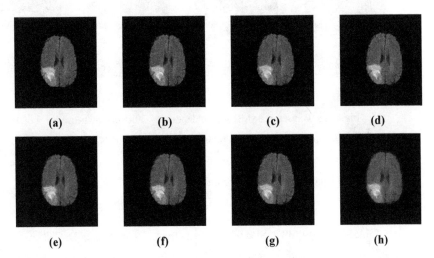

Fig. 3.17 Brain tumor MR image denoising with Poisson noise level of 15.
a) Original image b) Noisy image c) Pretrained DnCNN denoised images
d) Proposed DeepCNN denoised images e) Gaussian filter denoised images
f) Bilateral filter denoised images g) Adaptive filter denoised images
h) Guided filter denoised images.

Figure 3.18 shows the noise removal of brain tumor MR images, when the image is corrupted by known speckle noise level of 15. Original images and noisy images are shown in Fig. 3.18 a and b respectively. Here, the denoised images obtained by various models and filters like pretrained DnCNN model, proposed DeepCNN model, Gaussian filter, bilateral filter, adaptive filter, and guided filter are shown in Fig. 3.18 from c to h respectively. Among all filters and pertained DnCNN, the proposed DeepCNN provides better PSNR and SSIM in terms of performance. It is concluded that more PSNR and SSIM indicate that image has better quality.

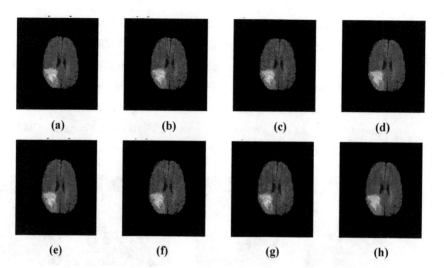

(a)   (b)   (c)   (d)

(e)   (f)   (g)   (h)

Fig. 3.18 Brain tumor MR image denoising with speckle noise level of 15.

a) Original image b) Noisy image c) Pretrained DnCNN denoised images

d) Proposed DeepCNN denoised images e) Gaussian filter denoised images

f) Bilateral filter denoised images g) Adaptive filter denoised images

h) Guided filter denoised images.

Table 3.3 PSNR (dB)/SSIM of proposed DeepCNN, pretrained DnCNN, Gaussian,
bilateral, adaptive, and guided filters for various noises with noise level 15.

S1. No	Noise Type / Filters	Gaussian		Poisson		Speckle		Salt and Pepper	
		PSNR	SSIM	PSNR	SSIM	PSNR	SSIM	PSNR	SSIM
1	DeepCNN	**22.39**	**0.1587**	**40.3205**	**0.98**	**39.4316**	**0.9705**	**19.6042**	0.2957
2	DnCNN	20.6564	0.1412	37.9084	0.9707	33.8085	0.9493	19.5151	0.2944
3	Gaussian Filter	17.3626	0.0581	36.6818	0.9593	28.9099	0.8918	19.2175	**0.3074**
4	Bilateral Filter	15.9876	0.0391	32.6595	0.9504	26.2759	0.8589	15.8919	0.2215
5	Adaptive Filter	19.0365	0.0698	37.4753	0.9618	27.2489	0.8783	17.7985	0.2483
6	Guided Filter	16.5214	0.0432	34.1424	0.9353	28.3088	0.8758	15.8473	0.2329
7	Median Filter	22.2424	0.1414	38.4352	0.9684	33.2793	0.9258	39.5647	0.9806

Table 3.3 presents the results of different filters on the addition of various noises with
noise level 15. The proposed DeepCNN model provides better PSNR and SSIM
values for the noisy image which is corrupted by known noise level of various noises.
In the table, the best results are marked in bold. The DeepCNN is not suitable for

reducing noise when the image is corrupted by salt and pepper noise with more than noise level 15. In case of reducing salt and pepper noise, the median filter is superior to all other filters and proposed method. Here higher values of SSIM indicated that the denoised image is structurally very close to original image. Due spatial filters, the PSNR, SSIM values are low for Gaussian and salt&pepper noise.

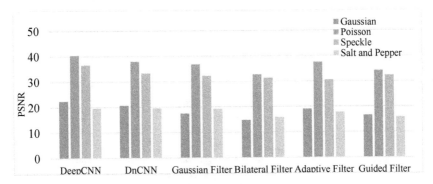

Fig. 3.19 PSNR performance comparison of various denoising methods.

Figure 3.19 shows the variation of PSNR in the form of a bar chart for the models (proposed DeepCNN and pretrained DnCNN) and four different filters (Gaussian filter (GAF), Bilateral filter (BF), Adaptive filter (AF), Guided filter (GUF)) with the addition of different noises like Gaussian, salt and pepper, Poisson and speckle noise. It can be observed that the proposed DeepCNN model gives better PSNR in dB of 40.3205, 39.4316, 22.39, and 19.6042 than that of pretrained DnCNN and other filters.

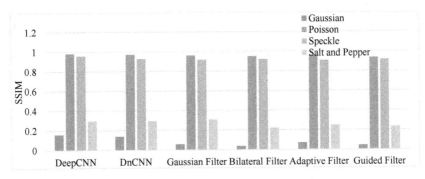

Fig. 3.20 SSIM performance comparison of various denoising methods.

Fig 3.20 shows the variation of SSIM in the form of a bar chart for the models (proposed DeepCNN and pretrained DnCNN) and four different filters (Gaussian filter (GAF), Bilateral filter (BF), Adaptive filter (AF), Guided filter (GUF)) with the addition of different noises like Gaussian, salt and pepper, Poisson and speckle noise. It can be observed that the proposed DeepCNN model gives better SSIM values of 0.98, 0.9705, 0.2957, and 0.1587 compared to that of pretrained DnCNN and other filters.

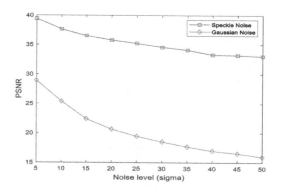

Fig. 3.21 PSNR (dB) performance comparison of proposed DeepCNN for Gaussian and speckle noise.

Figure 3.21 shows the PSNR in dB performance comparison of proposed DeepCNN for denoising of image corrupted with either Gaussian or speckle noise. It can be concluded from Fig. 3.21 that when the proposed DeepCNN model performs denoising of images corrupted with speckle and Gaussian noises of specified noise level 15, the DeepCNN is able to handle speckle noise very well.

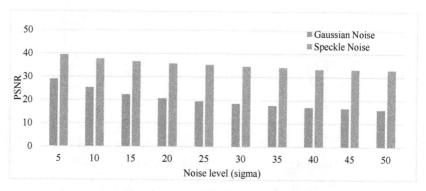

Fig. 3.22 PSNR (dB) performance comparison of proposed DeepCNN for Gaussian and speckle noise.

Figure 3.22 shows the variation of PSNR (dB) in the form of a bar chart for the Gaussian and speckle noise addition with noise level varying from 5 to 50. It can be observed that the PSNR in dB is improved by the proposed deepCNN for speckle noise compared to than that of Gaussian noise.

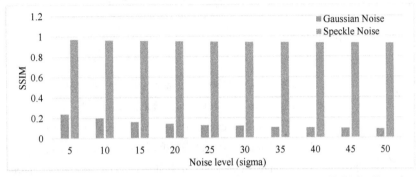

Fig. 3.23 SSIM performance comparison of proposed DeepCNN for Gaussian and speckle noise.

Fig 3.23 shows the variation of SSIM in the form of a bar chart for the Gaussian and speckle noise addition with noise level varying from 5 to 50. It can be observed that the SSIM value is improved by the proposed deepCNN for speckle noise compared to than that of Gaussian noise.

3.8 Conclusions

The performance of PSNR for Gaussian noise corrupted image is improved to 14.24 % with the proposed DeepCNN model for a noise level of 5. An improved performance of 7.66 % is achieved by the proposed model when speckle noise with an addition of noise level 5 is taken. For a Gaussian noise with known noise level of 15, the proposed DeepCNN model shows an improvement of PSNR by 8.39 %. Hence, the proposed DeepCNN model appears to be better for reducing noise when image gets corrupted by either speckle or Gaussian noise with known or unknown noise levels. In addition, the proposed DeepCNN preserves the structural information of the image by observing the SSIM values from the results. Classification of brain tumor MR images in to either LGG (benign) or HGG (malignant) using transfer learning and hybrid models are discussed in the next chapter.

Chapter 4

Brain Tumor MR Image Classification using Transfer Learning

4.1 Introduction

Human life is threatened by brain tumors and the chance of a patient's survival (Suter Y et al., 2018) increases, if it is being detected at an early stage. In recent years several studies have been conducted and it became a vital job to detect tumors in the brain via MR images (Kleihues P et al., 2000, Louis D N et al., 2016, Travis W D et al., 2015). A brain tumor arises when the brain develops a form of abnormal cells from inside. The two main forms of tumors: benign and malignant or cancerous tumors. Depending on the part of brain involved and symptoms they produce, the types of brain tumors may differ. These consist of symptoms like headaches, seizures, vision problems, vomiting, and mental changes.

As per the World Health Organization (WHO), the four kinds of tumors are: i) Grade I tumors are benign, slow-growing, and have long-term survival, ii) Grade II tumors are slow-growing relatively but at times recur as higher grade tumors, and are either benign or malignant. iii) Grade III tumors are malignant and frequently recur as higher grade tumors. iv) Grade IV tumors are violent, malignant tumors which grow rapidly. Among the various imaging techniques, brain magnetic resonance imaging (MRI) is one among the best options that researchers rely on for detecting the brain tumors and also to model the progression of tumor in detection as well as the treatment phases. Convolutional Neural Networks (CNNs) are the special case of neural network which provided major breakthroughs in many areas of image recognition and classification (Omer R and Liping F, 2010).

This chapter highlights how the pretrained models can be trained to small and different new data with SGDM (stochastic gradient decent with momentum) and ADAM (adaptive moment estimation) optimizers for classification task. Numerous hybrid models were proposed for the purpose of classifying the brain tumor MR image into benign or malignant tumor. The performance of the proposed models is evaluated in terms of accuracy, error rate, sensitivity, specificity, and F1-Score. This chapter is structured as follows. Section 4.2 presents overview of Artificial Neural Network including forward, back propagation process. Section 4.3 gives complete details of the convolutional neural networks. Various optimization methods used to minimize the loss function in CNN are discussed in the section 4.4. Section 4.5 introduces transfer learning approach for classification task, focuses on proposed methodologies and proposed models architectures for classification task. Section 4.6 discusses the performance metrics used for performance evaluation of the proposed models. Section 4.7 deals with experimental results and discussion. Finally, the conclusions are presented in section 4.8.

4.2 Introduction to Artificial Neural Network (ANN)

It has been some time since the CPUs have outraced human brain in terms of complex operations per second, for example, the floating point tasks. A single average CPU core processes in excess of 5 billion floating point operations (5 GFLOPS) which is very difficult for a human. Albeit human brain can't compute complex numerical operations, it can do considerably more than a CPU by consolidating numerous simple operations is as yet thought to be progressively effective tasks like image classification. So as to accomplish such tasks utilizing PCs, researchers have attempted to mimic the brain since 1940s and an idea called artificial neural networks has been developed.

4.2.1 Basics of Artificial Neural Networks

Artificial neurons are imitations of biological neurons. As shown in Fig. 4.1, a biological neuron produces an electrical signal. In the event that its dendrites are energized by sufficient number of synapses of other neurons, at that point it creates an electrical signal transmitted through its axon and energizes dendrites of different neurons through its synapse. Similar to the biological neurons, artificial neurons (or perceptron in its simpler form) are associated with one another and energize each other through these connections. They are capable of calculating only a very simple function called as neuron activation (Eq. 4.1). An artificial neuron was first proposed by W. McCulloch and W. Pitts in 1943 and shown in Fig. 4.2. It generates a binary output according to the result of this function and is called a perceptron (F Rosenblatt, 1958).

Fig. 4.1 shows how a biological neuron is fired when there is sufficient excitation by other connected neurons. Connections from one layer to the next have associated weights that tell the network how heavily a neuron's output should be considered, as seen in Fig. 4.2.

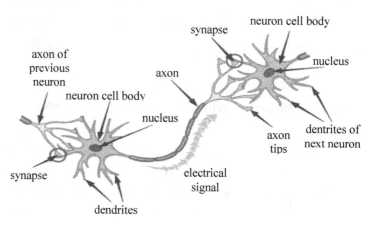

Fig. 4.1 Biological neuron.

$$a = \sum_{j=1}^{N} u_j w_j + b \qquad (4.1)$$

Here, u_j is an input layer, w_j is weights of the filters, b is bias, and a is a neuron in the layer, which will be activated later by an activation function.

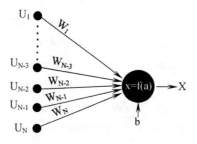

Fig. 4.2 Artificial neuron

72

If f(a) (activation function) is a threshold function, then the neuron is known as a perceptron. As the name suggests, an ANN is a network consisting of artificial neuron units having connections in between.

Feedforward networks: If the neurons are connected only in a single direction, the network is termed as a feedforward network i.e., a neuron cannot be connected to itself or another neuron which is closer to input. Formally, the outputs of $(n-1)^{th}$ layer are the inputs for n^{th} layer while n^{th} layer's outputs are inputs for $(n+1)^{th}$ layer. Connections between neurons that are in the same layer or that are in nonconsecutive layers are not permitted in feedforward neural networks. Fig. 4.3 shows an example of feedforward networks. Besides, a feedforward neural network having more than one hidden layers is called a deep neural network.

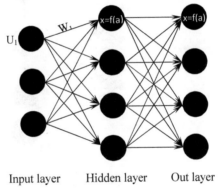

Input layer   Hidden layer   Out layer

Fig. 4.3   Feedforward neural network having one hidden layer

4.2.2 Multilayer networks

If there are at least one or more hidden layers, such a network is called Multilayer network. A single layer network by combining multiple neurons is given in Fig. 4.4 and Eq. 4.2 gives the input-output relation. Each neuron has its own bias and is not shown in Fig. 4.4. Eq. 4.3 gives the relation between input and output which is represented in a matrix form in in order to make the calculations simpler and the biases are merged into U and W matrices. A stack of single layers of neurons with the outputs connected to the inputs of another layer a multilayer network is obtained and is shown in Fig. 4.3.

$$x_i = f\left(\sum_{j=1}^{N} u_j w_{ji} + b\right) \tag{4.2}$$

73

$$X = f(W^T U) \qquad (4.3)$$

Where,

$$X = \begin{bmatrix} x_1 \\ x_2 \\ \vdots \\ x_M \end{bmatrix}, \ U = \begin{bmatrix} u_1 \\ u_2 \\ \vdots \\ u_N \\ 1 \end{bmatrix}, \ W = \begin{bmatrix} w_{01} & w_{02} & \cdots & w_{0M} \\ w_{11} & w_{12} & \cdots & w_{1M} \\ w_{21} & w_{22} & \cdots & w_{2M} \\ \cdots & \cdots & \cdots & \cdots \\ w_{N1} & w_{N2} & \cdots & w_{NM} \end{bmatrix}, \ B = \begin{bmatrix} b_{01} \\ b_{02} \\ \vdots \\ b_{0M} \end{bmatrix} \qquad (4.4)$$

Where, X is the output vector, U is the input vector, W is the weight matrix where the first row is equal to bias vector B.

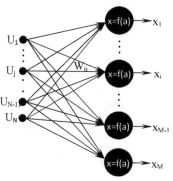

Fig. 4.4   Single layer network.

Generally, the accuracy of a neural network is improved by minimizing the loss function or cost function or error function, where weights, feed forward and back propagation process are used to optimize the biases. Various loss functions, activation functions, and optimization functions will be explained in optimization with back propagation in CNN section 4.4 because these are all approximately same for ANN and CNN.

4.3 Convolutional Neural Networks (CNN)

The biological neural network has inspired the artificial neural networks. Similarly, convolutional neural networks are inspired by the animal visual system. Although CNNs have been used in the literature for some time, but were rarely used

74

because of i) Lack of data to train the network and ii) Long training time due to lack of process parallelization. With the increasing number of photographs being uploaded on the Internet every day, the first problem has been overcome by the researchers. The advances in GPU technology has solved the second problem. Due to its nature of being parallelizable, the architecture of GPUs is more convenient to human brain than CPUs. There are many simple cores in a GPU, and for example, an Intel i7 7700k has a clock speed of 4.2 GHz while an NVIDIA GTX 1060 has a clock speed of 1500 MHz. whereas GTX 1060 has 1280 cores while i7 has 4 cores. Like a human brain, more number of weaker cores are more suitable for neural networks.

4.3.1 Layers of CNNs

The neural networks have some general characteristics like optimization methods, loss functions, etc., and are shared by the CNNs. Some of the characteristics of CNNs are focused in this section. Defining a network architecture is the first step to create and train a new convolutional neural network. The details of CNN layers are explained in this section.

The network architecture varies depending on the types and number of layers included which in turn depend on the particular application or data. A softmax layer and a classification layer must be used if there are categorical responses, and for the continuous response, a regression layer must be used at the end of the network. If small number of grayscale image data is available, a smaller network with only one or two convolutional layers might be sufficient to learn. But a more complicated network having number of convolutional and fully connected layers is desirable for complex data having millions of colored images. The CNN architecture uses the following layers and order too.

4.3.1.1 Image Input Layer

The images are provided as input to a network by an image input layer and data normalization is applied. Size of an image is specified and it should be accepted by image input layer. The height, width, and the number of color channels of that image gives the size of an image. The number of channels is one for a grayscale image, and it is 3 for a color image.

4.3.1.2 Convolutional Layer

A 2D convolutional layer applies sliding convolutional filters to the input. The convolutional layer consists of various components (Murphy K P, 2012).

Filters and Stride

A neurons of a convolutional layer connect to the sub regions of input images or the outputs of the previous layer. It learns the features localized by these regions as the image is getting scanned. The convolution operation computes a dot product of the weights and the input for each region, and a bias term is then added. A filter consists of a set of weights and applied to a region in the image. Fig. 4.5 shows a 3×3 filter scanning through the input, lower map representing the input and the output represented by the upper map.

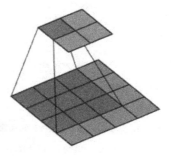

Fig. 4.5 Convolutional operation

A stride is the step size with which the filter is moved. Depending on the filter size and stride values, the local regions can overlap. The number of weights in a filter is $h \times w \times c$, where h, w, and c are the height, width of the filter, the number of channels in the input respectively. For a color image, there are three color channels and the number of channels in the output of a convolutional layer is determined by the number of filters.

Dilated Convolution

By specifying the dilation factor, the filters are expanded by inserting spaces between the elements of the filter. The dilated convolution is used to increase the receptive field (the area of the input which the layer can see) of the layer without increasing the number of parameters or computation. The filters are expanded by the layer using insertion of zeros between each filter element. The dilation factor is determined for sampling the input or equivalently the up-sampling factor of the filter and it corresponds to an effective filter size, $(\text{Filter Size-1}) \times \text{Dilation Factor} + 1$. A 3×3 filter with the dilation factor [2 2] is equivalent to 5×5 filter with zeros between the elements. The image in Fig. 4.5 shows a 3×3 filter dilated by a factor two, scanning through the input. The lower map represents the input and the output represented by the upper map.

Feature Maps

A filter uses the same set of weights and the same bias for the convolution while moving along the input, and forms a feature map as shown in Fig. 4.6. The number of feature maps is equal to the number of filters as each feature map is the result of a convolution and so the convolutional layer contains a total number of parameters $((\text{h} \times \text{w} \times \text{c} + 1) \times \text{Number of Filters})$, where bias is 1.

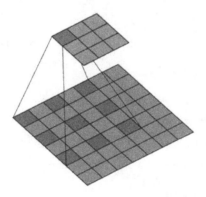

Fig. 4.6 Dilated convolutional operation

Zero Padding

A zero padding is the addition of rows or columns to the borders of an input image. The layer output size is controlled by adjusting the padding. The Fig. 4.7 shows a 3×3 filter which scans the input with padding of size 1. The input is represented by the lower map and the output by the upper map.

Output Size

The convolutional layer output has a height and width as

$$\frac{\text{(Input size} - \text{((filter size} - 1) \times \text{Dilation Factor} + 1) + 2 \times \text{padding}}{\text{stride}} + 1 \qquad (4.5)$$

For the whole image to be fully covered, the above value must be an integer.

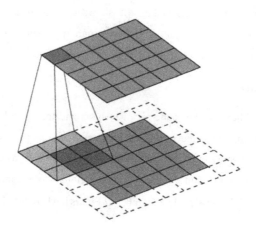

Fig. 4.7 Zero padding operation

Number of Neurons

The product of height and width of the output gives the total number of neurons in a feature map, i.e., the Map Size. The total number of neurons (output size) in a convolutional layer is Size × Number of Filters. Generally, the results from these neurons pass through some form of nonlinearity, such as rectified linear units (ReLU).

Learning Parameters

There is a provision of adjusting the learning rates and regularization options for the layer, by either defining the convolutional layer or training the network using training options.

Number of Layers

A convolutional neural network consists of one or multiple convolutional layers and the number of convolutional layers depends on the amount and complexity of the data.

4.3.1.3 Batch Normalization Layer

Each input channel across a mini-batch is normalized by a batch normalization layer (Ioffe S and C Szegedy et al., 2015). The training of convolutional neural networks is speed up and the sensitivity to network initialization is reduced by using batch normalization layers between convolutional layers and nonlinearities, such as ReLU layers. Activations of each channel are first normalized using this layer by subtracting the mini-batch mean and dividing the mini-batch standard deviation. Then, input is shifted by the layer using a learnable offset β and scaling by a learnable scale factor γ. The learnable parameters β and γ are updated during network training.

The normalization of the activations and gradients makes the network training an easier optimization problem. As the optimization problem is easier, the parameter updates can be larger and the network can learn faster. Also, the L_2 and dropout regularization can be reduced. To take full advantage of this regularizing effect, the training data can be shuffled before every training epoch.

4.3.1.4 ReLU Layer

Each element of the input is applied with a threshold operation using a ReLU layer (Nair V and G E Hinton, 2010) i.e., any value less than zero is set to zero. A nonlinear activation function follows Convolutional and batch normalization layers. The threshold operation is given as,

$$f(x) = \begin{cases} x, & x \geq 0 \\ 0, & x < 0 \end{cases} \tag{4.6}$$

The size of its input is not changed by the ReLU layer. There are other nonlinear activation layers that improve the network accuracy for some applications by performing different operations.

Cross Channel Normalization (local response normalization) Layer

The channel-wise normalization is done by a channel-wise local response (cross-channel) layer. It usually follows the ReLU activation layer and replaces each element with a normalized value that is obtained using the elements from a certain number of neighboring channels. For each element, x in the input, train network computes a normalized value x' as

$$x' = \frac{x}{(K+\frac{\alpha * ss}{window\,ChannelSize})^{\beta}} \qquad (4.7)$$

Where, K, α, and β are the hyper parameters, and the sum of squares of the elements in the normalization window (Krizhevsky A et al., 2012) is represented by ss.

4.3.1.5 Pooling Layers

A max pooling layer (Nagi J et al., 2011) executes down-sampling by dividing the input into rectangular pooling regions, and maximum of each region is computed. The input is divided into rectangular pooling regions and average values of each region are computed by using an average pooling layer. The convolutional layers are followed by the pooling layers for down-sampling, and so the number of connections to the following layers are reduced. They do not perform any learning themselves, but the number of parameters to be learned are reduced in the following layers. They also help to reduce over fitting.

4.3.1.6 Dropout Layer

It makes the elements to become zero randomly with a given probability. This is done at the training time, as given by the dropout mask. The underlying network architecture between iterations is effectively changed by this operation to help preventing the network from over-fitting (Srivastava N et al., 2014). A higher number results in more elements being dropped during training. The output of the layer is equal to its input at prediction time. No learning takes place in this layer just like in the max or average pooling layers.

4.3.1.7 Fully Connected Layer

The input is multiplied by a weight matrix W and then a bias vector b is added by the fully connected layer. One or more fully connected layers follow the convolutional (and down-sampling) layer. As per the name, all the neurons in the previous layer are connected to all neurons in a fully connected layer. It combines all of the features (local information) learned by the previous layers across the image to identify the larger patterns. Classification of images is done by combining the features of last fully connected layer. Therefore, the output size of the last fully connected layer of the network is equal to the number of classes of the dataset. The output size must be equal to the number of response variables for regression problems. The learning rate and the regularization parameters are adjusted for this layer, when the fully connected layer is created. If they are not adjusted here, they can be adjusted in training options while training the network.

4.3.1.8 Output Layers

Softmax and Classification layers are used for classification task and Regression layer is used for regression task.

Softmax and Classification Layers

The cross entropy loss is computed by a classification layer for multi-class classification problems with mutually exclusive classes. A softmax layer and then a classification layer must follow the final fully connected layer for classification problems. The output unit activation function is the softmax function:

$$y_r(x) = \frac{\exp(a_r(x))}{\sum_{j=1}^{k} \exp(a_j(x))} \qquad (4.8)$$

Where, $0 \leq y_r \leq 1$ and $\sum_{j=1}^{k} y_j = 1$

The classification layer must follow the softmax layer for typical classification network. In the classification layer, train network takes the values from the softmax function and each input to one of the K mutually exclusive classes are assigned using the cross entropy function for a one of k coding scheme (Bishop C. M, 2006):

$$loss = - \sum_{i=1}^{N} \sum_{j=1}^{K} t_{ij} \ln y_{ij} \qquad (4.9)$$

Where, N is the number of samples, K is the number of classes, t_{ij} is the indicator that the ith sample belongs to the jth class, and y_{ij} is the output for sample i for class j, which in this case, is the value from the softmax function.

Regression Layer

The half Mean Squared Error (MSE) loss is computed by a regression layer. For typical regression problems, the final fully connected layer must be followed by a regression layer. The mean squared error for a single observation is given by:

$$MSE = \sum_{i=1}^{R} \frac{(t_i \text{-} y_i)^2}{R}$$ (4.10)

Where, t_i is the target output, R is the number of responses and y_i is the network's prediction for response i. The loss function of the regression layer for image and sequence to one regression networks, is the half Mean Squared Error of the predicted responses, not normalized by R:

$$Loss = \frac{1}{2}\sum_{i=1}^{R} (t_i \text{-} y_i)^2$$ (4.11)

4.3.2 Activation Functions

For an activation function f(), the input of an artificial neuron is multiplied with the weights and is summed to a scalar to get the result as shown in Fig. 4.2. This section discusses the advantages and disadvantages of different activation functions.

Softmax

For the classification task of multilayer neural networks, softmax function (Eq. 4.6) is generally used in the output layer. The probability of each class is actually calculated using this function. This results in an output layer whose value equals to 1 which is sum of all softmax. Softmax estimates the more likely class to which the input belongs to instead of choosing between the classes. Softmax representation for an assumption of M classes is given as:

$$softmax(x_k) = \frac{e^{x_k}}{\sum_{i=1}^{M} e^{x_k}}$$ (4.12)

Sigmoid

Sigmoid function is restricted between 0 and 1. The main disadvantage is that, either for too large or too small values its gradients start to vanish. Further, as the values pass away from 0 and gets saturated the training gets slower (LeCun Y, Boser B et al., 1990). Sigmoid function is expressed as given below Eq. 4.13.

$$\text{sigmod}(x) = \frac{1}{1+e^{-x}} \tag{4.13}$$

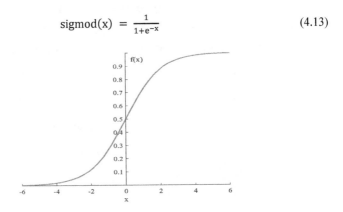

Fig. 4.8 Sigmoid function

Tanh function

The tanh function (Eq. 4.14, Fig. 4.11) is in general analogous to a sigmoid function but it is restricted between -1 and 1 instead of being restricted between 0 and 1. The tanh function is given in Eq. 4.14.

$$\tanh(x) = 2 \times \text{sigmoid}(x) - 1 = \frac{1-e^{-x}}{1+e^{-x}} \tag{4.14}$$

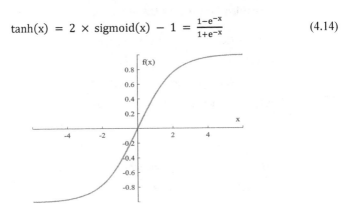

Fig. 4.9 Tanh function

Rectified Linear Unit (ReLU)

In neural networks, the functions that are nonlinear, differentiable, and symmetric were believed to be used better until the publishing of LeCun Y, Boser B et al., 1990. However, it has been shown that training a neural network can be made faster and computationally more efficient using rectified linear units (ReLU). The gradient descent (Eq. 4.15) can be easily computed for ReLUs as it is being differentiable everywhere except 0. On the other hand, at 0, its derivative is recognized and defined by the user as either 0 or 1. Moreover, for very large values the gradients does not vanish because the function does not saturate. So, the training is faster. Expression of ReLU is given in Eq. 4.15.

$$\text{ReLU} = \max(0,x) \tag{4.15}$$

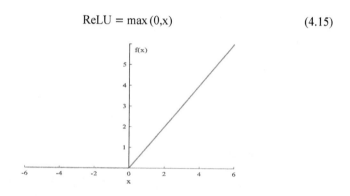

Fig. 4.10   ReLU function

Leaky Rectified Linear Unit (LReLU)

Leaky Rectified linear units results in a 0 output and gradient is 0 for any negative valued input as negative input values are somewhat ignored. Leaky rectified linear units (LReLU) are used to avoid the dying problem to have a constant gradient. In LReLUs, the function can be expressed as

$$\text{Leaky ReLU} = \max(\alpha x, x) \tag{4.16}$$

Where, α is a positive constant which is less than 1. It must be noted that for a trainable α value, the function is called parametric rectified linear unit (PReLU).

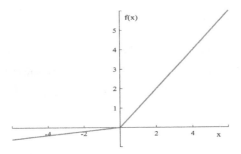

Fig. 4.11 Leaky ReLU function

4.4 Optimization with back propagation in neural networks

In neural networks, optimization is a vital part which updates the weights of neurons. Assuming a network with input u, output x, and let the target output (or the ground truth) is 't'. The weights are updated in the network using x = t. To do so, a cost function such as mean square error is introduced first. Mean square error for an assumption of N number of samples is given in Eq. 4.17.

$$\varepsilon = \frac{1}{N} \times \sum_{j=1}^{N} (t_j - x_j)^2 u \qquad (4.17)$$

To minimize Eq. 4.15, there exist several optimization methods. Newton's method is generally adapted to find the roots of a function by using the second order derivative. The computational complexity is increased significantly when compared to gradient descent method (H Robbins and S Monro, 1951, J Kiefer and J Wolfowitz, 1952) that use first order derivative. Because of this reason, gradient descent is chosen for training most neural networks.

Initial Weights and Biases

Gaussian distribution with a mean value of 0 and a standard deviation of 0.01is taken as default for choosing the initial weights. The default value for the initial bias is 0. The initialization for the weights and biases can be manually changed.

4.4.1 Optimizers

In this section, some optimizers like Stochastic Gradient Descent, Stochastic Gradient Descent with Momentum, Root Mean Square Propagation (RMSProp), and Adaptive moment estimation (ADAM) are discussed.

4.4.1.1 Stochastic gradient descent

To minimize the loss function, the network parameters (weights and biases) at each iteration are updated in the standard gradient descent algorithm by taking small steps in the direction of the negative of the loss gradient,

$$w_{i+1} = w(i) + \Delta w_i \tag{4.18}$$

$$\Delta w_i = -\mu \nabla \varepsilon(w_i) \tag{4.19}$$

$$\nabla \varepsilon(w_i) = \frac{\partial \varepsilon}{\partial w(i)} \tag{4.120}$$

$$x_j = w_j(i) u_j \tag{4.21}$$

$$\nabla \varepsilon(w_i) = \frac{\partial(\frac{1}{n} \times \sum_{j=1}^{n}(t_j - w_j(i) u_j)^2)}{\partial w(i)} \tag{4.22}$$

$$\nabla \varepsilon(w_i) = -\frac{2}{n} \times \sum_{j=1}^{n}(t_j - x_j) u_j \tag{4.23}$$

Where, i is the iteration number, learning rate is $\mu > 0$, loss function is $\varepsilon()$ and the weight matrix is w(i). The gradient of the loss function, $\nabla \varepsilon(w_i)$, is estimated in the standard gradient descent algorithm by the entire training set and the algorithm uses the entire data set at once.

In contrast, the stochastic gradient descent algorithm estimates the gradient at each iteration and a subset of the training data updates the parameters. At each iteration, a different subset known as mini-batch is used. One epoch uses mini-batches of the training algorithm over the entire training set for the full pass. Stochastic gradient descent is stochastic because by using a mini-batch the parameter updates a computed noisy estimate of the parameter that would update the result from using the full data set.

The gradient descent starts to oscillate in some dimensions as it approaches to the minimum and is as shown in Fig. 4.12. After each iteration these dimensions may change since gradient direction due to the noise exhibited from samples (R S Sutton, 1986).

Momentum

The oscillations specified above may be decreased by adding a parameter called momentum as shown in Fig. 4.12. Refining the classical gradient descent Eq 4.19, the update with momentum converts to Eq. 4.24 (D E Rumelhart, 1986, N Qian, 1999).

$$\Delta w_i = \delta \nabla w_{i-1} - \mu \nabla \varepsilon(w_i) \tag{4.24}$$

Where, δ is momentum parameter.

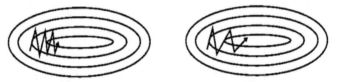

Fig. 4.12 Left is gradient descent without momentum, right is the gradient descent with momentum.

4.4.1.2 Stochastic gradient descent with momentum

This oscillation can be reduced by adding a momentum term to the parameter update and the stochastic gradient descent algorithm can oscillate towards the optimum along the path of steepest descent. The update for stochastic gradient descent with momentum (SGDM) is

$$w_{i+1} = w_i + \Delta w_i \tag{4.25}$$

$$w_{i+1} = w_i - \mu \nabla \varepsilon(w_i) + \delta(w_i - w_{i-1}) \tag{4.26}$$

Where, δ denotes the contribution of the previous gradient step to the current iteration.

4.4.1.3 Root Mean Square Propagation (RMSProp)

A single learning rate is used for all the parameters in stochastic gradient descent algorithm with momentum. To improve network training, other optimization algorithms try to use learning rates differing by parameter and automatically adapts to the loss function being optimized. RMSProp (root mean square propagation) is such an algorithm keeping the parameter gradients as a moving average of the element wise squares.

$$v_l = \beta_2 v_{l-1} + (1-\beta_2) \left[\nabla\varepsilon(w_i)\right]^2 \tag{4.27}$$

Where, β_2 is the decay rate of the moving average. The common values used for decay rate are 0.9, 0.99, and 0.999. For squared gradients, the corresponding averaging lengths equal, $1/(1-\beta_2)$ that is, 10, 100, and 1000 parameter updates, respectively. Individually, the updates of each parameter uses this moving average to normalize the RMSProp algorithm as

$$w_{i+1} = w_i - \frac{\alpha\nabla\varepsilon(w_i)}{\sqrt{v_l}+\gamma} \tag{4.28}$$

Where, element-wise division is made. The learning rates of parameters effectively decreases with large gradients using RMSProp and with small gradients the learning rates of parameters increases. To avoid division by zero, a small constant γ is added.

4.4.1.4 Adaptive moment estimation (ADAM)

ADAM (LeCun Y et al., 1998) that is similar to RMSProp uses a parameter update but with an added momentum term. It preserves both the parameter gradients and their squared values by moving average of element-wise values,

$$m_l = \beta_1 m_{l-1} + (1-\beta_1)\nabla\varepsilon(w_i) \tag{4.29}$$

$$v_l = \beta_2 v_{l-1} + (1-\beta_2)[\nabla\varepsilon(w_i)]^2 \tag{4.30}$$

Where, β_1 and β_2 decay rates are gradient decay factor and squared gradient decay factor respectively. To update the network parameters, ADAM uses the moving averages as

$$w_{i+1} = w_i - \frac{\alpha m_l}{\sqrt{v_l} + \varepsilon} \tag{4.31}$$

For all optimization algorithms, α is specified as the initial learning rate. Different optimization algorithms have different effect of the learning rate. So, in general the optimal learning rates are also different.

4.4.2 Back propagation

Due to high number of unknowns in a neural network the optimization task turns out to be more complex and thus there can be numerous neurons that have many weights. The process of error propagation from output to input using the chain rule, (Y. LeCun et al., 1998) is called backpropagation.

An equation using backpropagation is found for each weight to have same number of equations, unknowns and by propagating error through the input this is done. Then, according to the weights the derivative of those propagated errors is calculated correspondingly. To find the change in output x_k the backpropagation on a multilayer network is performed by applying the chain rule with respect to weight of jth input of ith neuron in L^{th} layer $w_{L,j,i}$. Fig. 4.7 shows the applied structure starting from the output layer using the chain rule. With Eq. 4.5, a single output x_k can be represented in terms of the weights in the last layer and the previous layer outputs are as shown in equation 4.32.

$$x_k = f(W_{(L+1),k}^T x_L) \tag{4.32}$$

Where, f( ) is an activation function. In the hidden layer, the output of a neuron can also be represented as in equation 4.33.

$$x_{L,i} = f\left(W_{L,i}^T u\right) \tag{4.33}$$

In order to use gradient descent to $w_{L,j,i}$, $\frac{\partial \varepsilon}{\partial w_{L,j,i}}$ is required. ε is the MSE as specified in Eq. 4.17. Equation 4.34 can be found by applying chain rule.

$$\frac{\partial \varepsilon}{\partial w_{L,j,i}} = \frac{\partial \varepsilon}{\partial x_k} \frac{\partial x_k}{\partial w_{L,i,j}} \tag{4.34}$$

$$\frac{\partial x_k}{\partial w_{L,j,i}} = \frac{\partial x_k}{\partial x_{L,i}} \frac{\partial x_{L,i}}{\partial w_{L,i,j}} \tag{4.35}$$

89

$$\frac{\partial \varepsilon}{\partial w_{L,j,i}} = \frac{\partial \varepsilon}{\partial x_k} \frac{\partial x_k}{\partial x_{L,i}} \frac{\partial x_{L,i}}{\partial w_{L,i,j}} \tag{4.36}$$

Which, using equations 4.32 and 4.33, becomes equation 4.37

$$\frac{\partial \varepsilon}{\partial w_{L,j,i}} = -\frac{2}{M} \times (t_k - x_k) f'(W_{(L+1),k}^T x_L) w_{(L+1),i,k} f'(W_{L,i}^T u) u_i \tag{4.37}$$

However, all of the weights $w_{(L+1),j,k}$ is affected when backward, $w_{L,j,i}$ is propagated where k varies from 1 to M. Thus, by adding these partial derivatives, Eq. 4.38 is obtained.

$$\frac{\partial \varepsilon}{\partial w_{L,j,i}} = -\frac{2}{M} \times \sum_{k=1}^{M} (t_k - x_k) f'(W_{(L+1),k}^T x_L) w_{(L+1),i,k} f'(W_{L,i}^T u) u_i \tag{4.38}$$

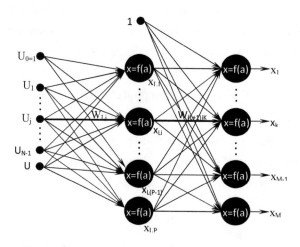

Fig. 4.13 Backpropagation of x_k for $w_{L,j,i}$

Solution of Eq. 4.38 is simple if the derivative of the activation function $f()$ calculation is easy. This is why activation functions like rectified linear function is preferred in neural networks.

4.4.3 Loss functions

Some of the loss functions available are mean squared error loss, mean squared logarithmic error loss, mean absolute error loss for regression loss functions; binary classification loss functions include binary cross entropy, hinge loss, squared hinge loss; loss functions of multi class classification problem are multi-class cross-entropy loss, sparse multiclass cross entropy loss; and dice similarity coefficient loss function is used as a loss function for image segmentation.

4.4.3.1 Mean Square Error (MSE) loss function

The performance is affected mainly by the error function used for the optimization as seen from Eq. 4.19 to Eq. 4.38. The Loss function selection depends on the task. For regression problems whose aim is to reach a continuous variable then mean square error (Eq. 4.17) or mean absolute error can be used. Similarly, error functions like cross entropy and likelihood loss are used in classification problems, where the target value is discrete (1 if belongs to that class, 0 otherwise). Specifically, for image segmentation problem a differentiable version of dice score can be used. Loss functions that can be used for the segmentation problem is given in detail based on the scope of this thesis.

4.4.3.2 Cross entropy loss function

The most extensively used cost function is cross entropy for image classification and image segmentation as given by Eq. 4.39 which is similar to mean square error that measures the distribution characteristics of two representations.

$$D(S,L) = - \sum_i^c L_i \log S_i \qquad (4.39)$$

Where, C is the number of classes, S is the predicted output (softmax output) and L is the ground truth label. The cross entropy is calculated for each pixel for segmentation case and reduced to a scalar. Basically one must consider both class members where $L_i=1$ and non-class members $L_i=1$ in order to turn this into a cost function. Thus, equation becomes Eq. 4.40.

$$D_{loss}(S,L) = - \sum_i^c L_i \log S_i - \sum_i^c (1-L_i) \log(1-S_i) \qquad (4.40)$$

Operations such as summation or averaging of each pixel can be used for the reduction purpose in image segmentation problems.

4.4.3.3 Weighted cross entropy

Eq. 4.41 can be used in order to solve the class imbalance problem, where W_i is the weight corresponding to i^{th} class that belongs to. W_i values can be selected inversely proportional to number of samples in i^{th} class.

$$D_{loss}(S,L) = -\sum_i^c W_i L_i \log S_i - \sum_i^c (1-L_i) \log(1-S_i) \tag{4.41}$$

4.4.3.4 Dice similarity coefficient loss function

For image segmentation, another loss function used is the dice loss function (Eq. 4.42). It is analogous to dice coefficient which is explained in section 6.3.1. The only difference is that instead of using sparse results, to calculate the dice coefficient softmax results are used so that it becomes differentiable. Note that, in BraTS 2017 challenge two of the top performing methods proposed used dice loss (K Kamnitsas et al., 2017, F Isensee et al., 2017).

$$Dice\ Loss = -\frac{2}{|C|} \sum_i^C \frac{\sum_k S_i^k L_i^k}{\sum_k S_i^k + \sum_k L_i^k} \tag{4.42}$$

Where, C is the number of classes and k is every pixel in the image.

4.5 Transfer Learning (TL)

To transfer knowledge between tasks of human learners seem to have inherent ways. That is, relevant knowledge is to be recognized and applied from earlier learning experience when new tasks are encountered. The more is the new task related to an earlier experience, the more easily it can be mastered.

The learning of a related target task can be improved by using transfer learning which includes the method in which knowledge is learnt in one or more source tasks used and transferred as shown in Fig. 4.14. The advance of algorithms that enable transfer learning while most deep learning algorithms are designed to address single tasks is a subject of current interest in the deep learning community.

Natural images trained on most of the deep neural networks show an interested phenomenon in common: they learn features on the first layer like color blobs and Gabor filters. That kind of first layer features are not certain to a particular dataset or task but are applicable to many datasets and tasks in general. Irrespective of the exact cost function and natural image dataset, these first-layer features are in general seems to occur as finding of these standard features on the first layer. For instance, these last-layer features are specific in a network with an N-dimensional softmax output layer that has been successfully trained towards a supervised classification objective, each output unit will be specific to a particular class.

In transfer learning, a base network is trained first on a base dataset, task, and then repurposed the learned features or transfer them, to a second target network to be trained on the target dataset and task. This process works well if the features are general, i.e., suitable to both base and target tasks, instead of being specific to the base task. In general, very few people train on an entire Convolutional Network from scratch and do it is quite rare to have a dataset of sufficient size. So, a CNN is generally pretrained on a very large dataset (e.g., ImageNet containing 1.2 million images having 1000 categories), and CNN is used either as an initialization or a fixed feature extractor for the task of interest.

Depending on the resemblance of the new dataset to the original dataset as well as size of the new dataset, the method of using transfer learning is different. In this thesis, the target dataset is small and different from the base training dataset for the purpose of classification. As the dataset is small, over-fitting is a concern. Hence, the linear layers are only trained. But as the base dataset is very much different from the target dataset, the higher-level features would not be of any relevance to the target dataset in CNN. Therefore, the new network uses only the low level features in the base CNN. The following steps are considered to implement this.

- Most of the pretrained layers are removed near the beginning of the CNN
- New fully connected layers are added to the remaining pretrained layers that match the number of classes in the new dataset.
- The new fully connected (dense) layer weights are randomized and all the weights are then freezed from the pretrained network.
- The network has to be trained to update the weights of the new fully connected layers.

4.5.1 Architecture of Alexnet

AlexNet (Krizhevsky Alex et al., 2012) is a state of the art image classification CNN Model and is given in Fig. 4.14 in order to show convolution, pooling, and fully connected layers. It is a total of 25 layers network and includes one input layer, 5 convolutional layers, 7 ReLU (activation function), 2 batch normalization layers, 3 max pooling layers, 3 fully connected layers (dense), 2 dropout layers, one softmax layer, one output layer (1000). First feature map is obtained by 96 convolutional filters of size $11 \times 11 \times 3$ are convolution with input image size of 227 pixels × 227 pixels × 3 channels with stride equal to 4 and padding 1. There are no up-sampling layers as it is a classification network. For segmentation case, the fully connected (dense) layers at the end become 1×1 convolutional layers. Various layers used in the model are discussed in this section and layer information along with the total number of learnable parameters trained are shown in Fig. 4.17.

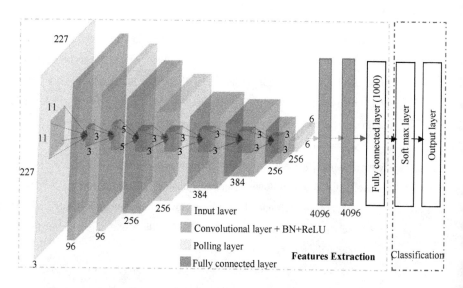

Fig. 4.14 Alexnet.

It has the capability of classifying 1000 classes because the output layer is having 1000 object categories. Some of the object categories of Alexnet are animals, flowers, pencil, mouse, tea cup, jug, keyboard, etc. As a result, the rich features are learned by Alexnet model to classify the classes for a wide range of images. Input image size of this model is 227 pixels × 227 pixels × 3 channels and Alexnet is also used directly to classify a new image. The model is trained to 61 million parameters and has 0.72 billion operations per prediction. Memory size of the Alexnet is 245 MB. In the ImageNet Large Scale Visual Recognition Challenge (ILSVRC) (Russakovsky et al., 2012), Alexnet stood as an outperformer with accuracy of 83.6 % and reduced the error rate from 26 % to 16.4 %.

4.5.2 TL method and methodology

Alexnet is one of the revolutionary pretrained convolutional neural network and trained on more than one million images from the ImageNet database. The layers of transfer learning model are connected to each other and shown in three dimensional view as shown in Fig. 4.16. First and third convolutional filters are of size 11 × 11 and 5 × 5 and remaining all convolutional filters are of size 3 × 3. The number of convolutional filters from first to last are 96, 96, 256, 256, 384, 384, 256, and 256 and next three layers are dense layers.

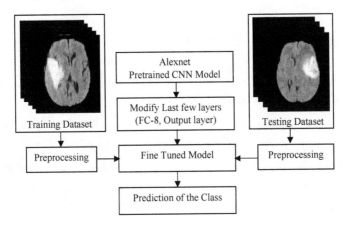

Fig. 4.15 Framework of transfer learning model (Fine tuning of Alexnet model).

To retain a pertained Alexnet model to predict new images of dataset, a few layers of this model have to be replaced with new layers and adjust according to the new images of dataset. The number of classes must be changed to match new images of dataset. The twenty third layer of the pretrained Alexnet, fully connected layer (fc8) should be replaced with new fully connected layer (newfc8) using parameters like output size to the number of classes in the new images of dataset (the number of

95

classes in this work are 2, benign and malignant) and learning rates are modified so that training process for new dataset is speeded up.

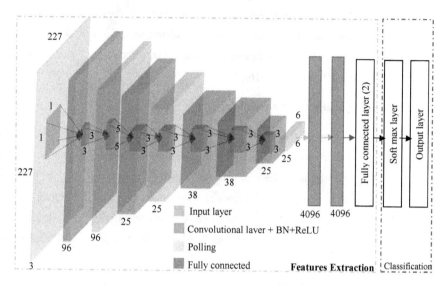

Fig. 4.16 Architecture of modified Alexnet (Transfer learning).

The learning rate parameters are weight learn rate factor and bias learn rate factor, both are set to 20. An original classification layer (output) should be replaced with new classification layer (newoutput). This new classification layer is also set to the number of classes i.e., 2. All these modifications can be seen in Fig. 4.16 and Fig. 4.18. Now transfer learning model is ready for training with dataset. In the next section, the preprocessing of training dataset, validation dataset, and testing dataset are discussed. The model is trained using training dataset and then classified the images for testing dataset.

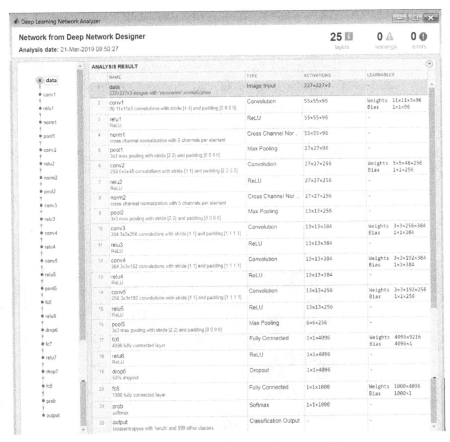

Fig. 4.17 An interactive visualization of Alexnet architecture.

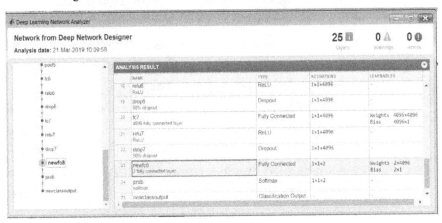

Fig. 4.18 Modified last three layers of transfer learning model.

97

4.5.3 TL features with ML classifier (Hybrid models)

The architecture of the hybrid CNN-KNN model is shown in Fig. 4.19 and Fig. 4.20, shows methodology of the proposed model, and its layers. The proposed methodology includes 25 layers out of which there are five Convolutional layers and the first layer is an input image of 227 pixels × 227 pixels × 3 channels with zero center normalization. The second layer is a convolutional layer which includes 96 convolutional filters with 11 × 11 × 3 size with stride 4 and zero padding is applied to the input image.

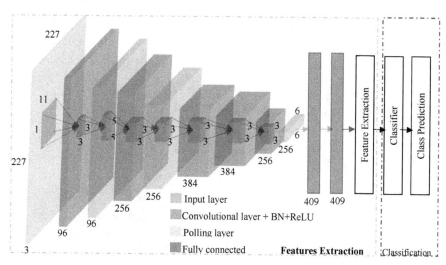

Fig. 4.19 Block diagram of proposed hybrid model.

In this stage, low level features such as edges, blobs, shapes, etc., are obtained. A nonlinear activation function, ReLU and cross channel normalization with five channels per element are applied to the previous convolutional layer 'conv1'. Downsampling is applied on this model by using a maxpooling layer of 3 × 3 with stride 2 and zero padding. The above discussion is for one convolutional block and the proposed model has five of such convolutional bocks. The second convolutional block is similar to the first convolutional block, but the convolutional layer is 256 filters of size 5 × 5 × 48 with stride 1 and padding 2. Third and fourth convolutional blocks are with 384 filters of size 3 × 3 and padding 1 and there is no maxpooling layer. The fifth block is similar to the first block except for having 256 convolutional filters. Then 3 fully connected layers are used to connect all the neurons in the layers.

50 % dropout layer is connected between the fully connected layers to make 50 % of neurons not activated. Last but one layer is softmax layer to evaluate the probability of class occurrence.

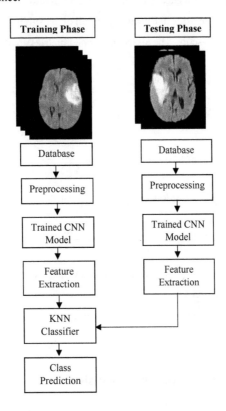

Fig. 4.20 Frame work of CNN-KNN image classification.

The different classes in this classification problem are benign and malignant. The last fully connected layer is modified as two class classification task having parameters, such as, bias learn rate factor and weight learn rate factor. From CNN, a highly representative features are extracted and then applied to various shallow machine learning classifiers like K-Nearest Neighbors (KNN), Discriminant (DISCR), Support Vector Machine (SVM), Naive Bayes (NB), Ensemble (ENSEMBLE), and Decision Tree (TREE) to classify the given brain tumor MR image in to either LGG case (benign) or HGG case (malignant).

4.6 Performance evaluation metrics

The proposed transfer learning model and hybrid models are evaluated based on the performance metrics like accuracy, recall or sensitivity, precision or specificity, error rate and the F1-score. The above mentioned metrics are defined as follows.

$$\text{Accuracy} = \frac{TP+TN}{TP+TN+FP+FN} \times 100 \qquad (4.43)$$

$$\text{Recall or Sensitivity} = \frac{TP}{TP+FN} \qquad (4.44)$$

$$\text{Precision or Specificity} = \frac{TN}{TN+FP} \qquad (4.45)$$

$$\text{Error Rate} = \frac{FP+FN}{TP+TN+FP+FN} \times 100 \qquad (4.46)$$

$$\text{F1- Score} = 2 \times \frac{\text{Specificity} \times \text{Sensitivity}}{\text{Specificity} + \text{Sensitivity}} \qquad (4.47)$$

Where, TP represents True Positive (malignant tumor is predicted correctly), TN is True Negative (benign tumor is predicted correctly), FP is False Positive (benign tumor is predicted as malignant tumor wrongly), and FN is False Negative (malignant tumor predicted as benign tumor wrongly).

4.7 Experimental results and discussion

In this section, the experimental results of brain tumor MR images classification using transfer learning model and hybrid models are discussed.

4.7.1 Brain tumor classification with TL model

Normally, selecting a data base is very difficult task for image denoising (Zhang Kai et al., 2017), segmentation and classification. A popular database for brain tumor images, BraTS 2018 database is considered to prepare various datasets like training, validation, and testing datasets. With 660 images including both benign and malignant tumor images, a new database is prepared and named as Brain Tumor Database-660 (BTD-660). In this BTD-660 database, 400 images of training dataset including 200 images of benign tumor and 200 images of malignant tumor cases,

100

testing dataset of 120 benign and 120 malignant tumor images. Validation dataset includes benign tumor images of 10 and malignant tumor images of 10.

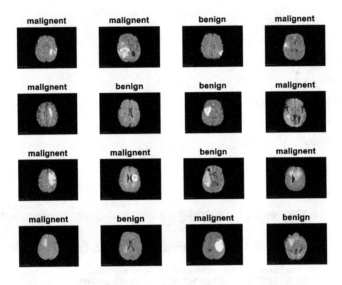

Fig. 4.21 Training images of 16 random images from training dataset.

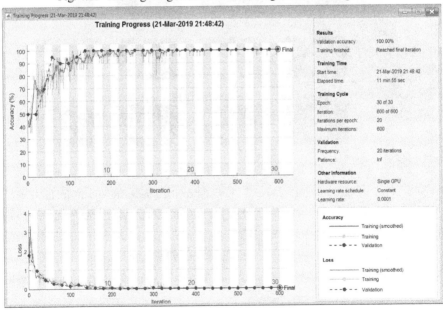

Fig. 4.22 Training process of transfer learning model.

Fig. 4.21, it is clear that there are 16 randomly selected brain tumor images of both classes benign and malignant tumors which are presented here from training dataset.

The transfer learning model is then trained to these datasets of training and validation datasets with training options like optimizer sets to either stochastic gradient descent with momentum (SGDM) or adaptive moment estimation (ADAM), mini batch size 20, max epochs 30, initial learning rate 0.0001, and validation frequency 20. The model is trained with an accuracy of 100 % and reached validation accuracy to 100 %. Remaining all the information related to training process is shown in Fig. 4.22.

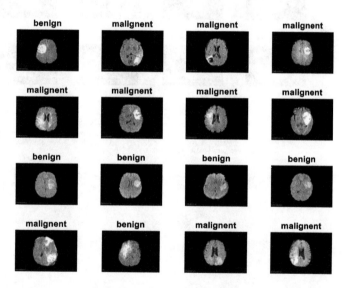

Fig. 4.23 Testing images of 16 random images from testing dataset.

Once training process is reached to the maximum epoch, it shows that the training process is completed. Now it's time to evaluate the trained model with testing dataset. Fig. 4.23, it is clear that there are 16 randomly selected brain tumor images of both classes benign and malignant tumors which are presented here from testing dataset.   Fig. 4.24 shows the proposed model is predicted the class of randomly selected 16 individual images in the testing dataset with predicted probability.

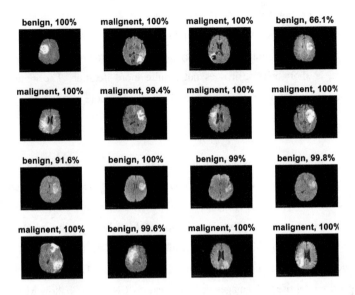

Fig. 4.24 Testing images of 16 random images with prediction percentage from testing dataset.

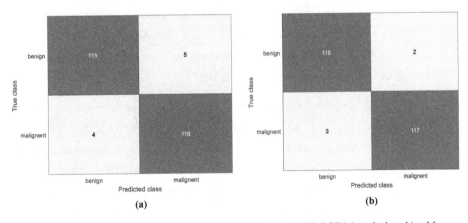

Fig. 4.25 Confusion matrices of proposed TL model a) with SGDM optimizer b) with ADAM optimizer.

Figure 4.25 shows the classification results of the proposed TL model with SGDM optimizer (left) and with ADAM optimizer (right) in terms of confusion matrix. The proposed transfer learning model is misclassified as 9 images out of 240 images, when SGDM is used as optimizer and five images are misclassified by the model, when ADAM is used as optimizer. From these confusion matrice, the performance matrices of the proposed model is evaluated. The model has following performance metrics, with SGDM optimizer accuracy is 96.25 %, error rate is 3.75 % and with ADAM optimizer accuracy is 97.91 %, error rate is 2.08 %. The training period is short because it does not require more iteration. The input weights and biases are both randomly generated as TL method is more efficient.

4.7.2 Brain tumor classification with Hybrid models

In this thesis, extraction of huge number of non-handcrafted i.e., high level complex representative features, is done using CNN model and then several classifiers are considered for classifying given MRI brain images into either of the two classes. Here various classifiers for classification of MRI brain tumors used are k Nearest Neighbors (KNN), Discriminant (DISCR), Support Vector Machine (SVM), Naive Bayes (NB), Ensemble (ENSEMBLE), and Decision Tree (TREE). The proposed hybrid model uses advantages of both methods CNN and Shallow Machine learning algorithms like KNN, DISCR), SVM, NB, ENSEMBLE, and TREE. For example, in the hybrid model CNN-KNN, the advantages of CNN are sparse connectivity among the neurons between successive layers and weights shared between layers. The nearest data samples are classified by the KNN as a class based on similar measures. The CNN-KNN model would have the combined salient features automatically and laborious and time consumption is reduced.

Evaluation of the proposed models is performed on the image database, BraTS 2018 and executed on Lenovo laptop with Intel i5, 7th generation processor, 8 GB DDR4 RAM, and 4GB NVIDIA graphics card. BraTS 2018 contains volumetric images, available in Low Grade Glioma (LGG) i.e., benign and High Grade Glioma (HGG) i.e., malignant. In the preprocessing, training and testing dataset are both processed in required format and used for training and testing phases. Each of the images has a size of 227 x 227 x 3 channels. The CNN model is trained with a training dataset of 400 images consisting of 200 benign and 200 malignant images. The architecture of the CNN model is described in CNN model architecture as shown in Fig. 4.19. At deeper level, high level features are extracted from fully connected layer using activation function. For each image, 4096 non-hand crafted features are extracted. In this way, 4096 non-hand crafted features of 400 images are then used to train the KNN classifier with specified training options.

On the other hand, the CNN model is trained by a testing dataset of 240 images which consists of 120 benign and 120 malignant images, and 4096 non hand-crafted features are extracted for each image. Then the classifier predicts the class of input image whether it is benign (LGG) or malignant (HGG). Finally, evaluation is done for the proposed CNN-KNN by finding the accuracy based on confusion matrix.

The Fig. 4.26 shows the training options of CNN-KNN model. Training of the model is done by using stochastic gradient descent momentum optimizer with 0.0001 learning rate. The model is trained for 30 epochs with mini-batch size of 20 images. Initially accuracy and loss of the mini-batch started with 60 % and 0.6910 and finally reached to 100 % and 0.0020 respectively.

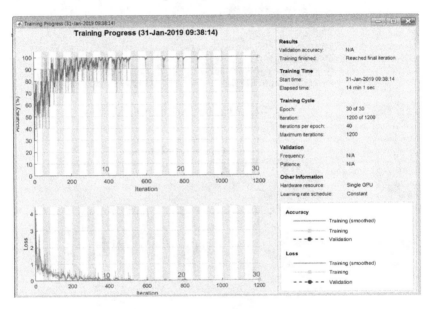

Fig. 4.26 Training options of CNN-KNN model.

The Low level features of the first convolutional layer and weights of 96 convolutional filters of size $11 \times 11 \times 3$ are shown in Fig. 4.28 and Fig. 4.27, respectively. These features are edges, blobs, and shapes, etc. Fig. 4.29 shows the second convolutional layer features, which are obtained from previous convolutional layer. The high level representative features of deeper layer, these features are obtained from previous convolutional layer 6. Features of fully connected layer 7 are

105

shown in Fig. 4.30. These features are then used as input to the classifiers to classify the given input image in to either benign or malignant

First convolutional layer weights

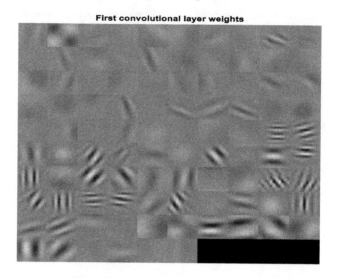

Fig. 4.27 Weights of first convolutional layer.

Layer conv1 Features

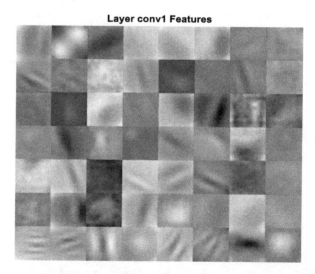

Fig. 4.28 Features of the first convolutional layer.

Layer conv2 Features

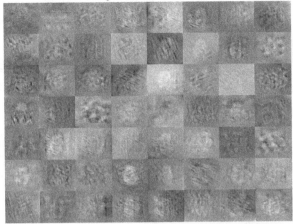

Fig. 4.29 Features of the second convolutional layer.

Layer fc7 Features

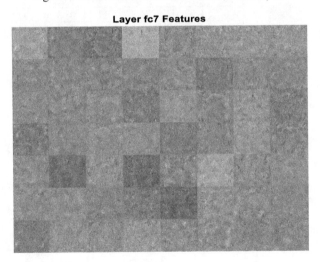

Fig. 4.30 Features of the fully connected (dense) layer.

Similarly, other hybrid models like CNN (built-in Classifier), CNN-Discriminant (CNN-DISCR), CNN-Support Vector Machine (CNN-SVM), CNN-Naive Bayes (CNN-NB), CNN-ESEMBLE, CNN-TREE follow the same procedures for training and testing phase. As discussed in section 4.7.2, among all hybrid models, the proposed CNN-KNN model is a promising model for MRI brain tumor classification. Experimental results of hybrid and TL models and their performance comparison are discussed in the next section 4.7.3.

4.7.3 Comparison of TL model with hybrid models

The performance parameters like accuracy, error rate, F1-score, sensitivity, and specificity evaluated for TL models are based on the confusion matrix obtained and are then compared with hybrid models. The transfer learning model with two optimizers ADAM and SGDM along with hybrid models are plotted and among the hybrid models, CNN-KNN show better performance whereas among the TL models, the TL model with ADAM optimizer shows the best performance.

Table 4.1 Confusion matrix of various classification models.

S.No	Method	TN	FP	FN	TP
1	TL with ADAM	118	2	3	117
2	TL with SGDM	115	5	4	116
3	CNN-KNN	116	4	5	115
4	CNN	117	3	7	113
5	CNN-DISCR	116	4	6	114
6	CNN SVM	115	5	7	113
7	CNN-NB	106	14	8	112
8	CNN-ENSEMBLE	106	14	9	111
9	CNN-TREE	102	18	11	109

Table 4.1 represents confusion matrices of various classification models like TL with ADAM, TL with SGDM, CNN-KNN, CNN, CNN-DISCR, CNN-SVM, CNN-NB, CNN-ENSEMBLE, and CNN-TREE. All these models are evaluated on a test data set of 240 images, out of which TL with ADAM optimizer shows the best result with only 5 images misclassified and also with least false negative (FN) of 3 images.

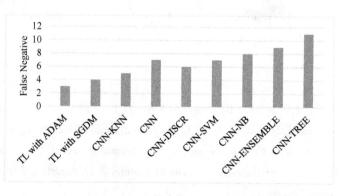

Fig. 4.31 Plot of false negative versus various classification models.

False negative case is considered to be the highest risk factor as malignant tumor is wrongly misclassified as benign and patient will be at high risk if neglected. So, above Fig. 4.31 is drawn for all the models for false negative cases. Hence TL with ADAM optimizer is shown to be the better model for reducing the misclassification of cancer cases.

Table 4.2 Performance comparison of various classification methods.

Sl. No	Method	Recall (or) Sensitivity	Precision (or) Specificity	F1 Score	Error Rate (%)	Accuracy (%)
1	TL with ADAM	**0.9750**	**0.9833**	**0.9791**	**2.08**	**97.92**
2	TL with SGDM	0.9667	0.9583	0.9625	3.75	96.25
3	CNN-KNN	0.9583	0.9667	0.9625	3.7500	96.25
4	CNN	0.9417	0.9750	0.9581	4.1666	95.83
5	CNN-DISCR	0.9500	0.9667	0.9582	4.1666	95.83
6	CNN-SVM	0.9417	0.9583	0.9499	5.0000	95.00
7	CNN-NB	0.9333	0.8833	0.9076	9.1666	90.83
8	CNN-ENSEMBLE	0.9250	0.8833	0.9037	9.5833	90.47
9	CNN-TREE	0.9083	0.8500	0.8782	12.0833	87.97

From Table 4.2, the true positive rate (recall or sensitivity) of the proposed TL model with ADAM optimizer is more, compared to all other methods. Among all these methods, the proposed TL with ADAM shows better performance like accuracy of 97.92 % and F1 score of 0.9791. With least error rate of 2.08 %, the proposed TL with ADAM optimizer is the best model out of all the models.

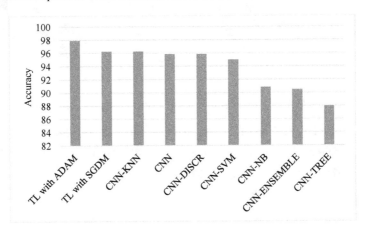

Fig. 4.32 Plot of accuracy versus various classification models.

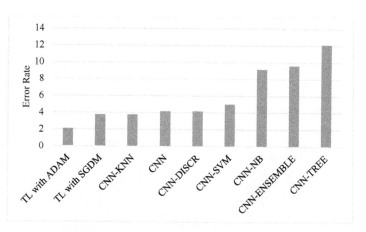

Fig. 4.33 Plot of error rate versus various classification models.

Fig. 4.32 and Fig. 4.33 show the bar chart for accuracy and error rate of various models and it is clear that TL with ADAM optimizer has good accuracy of 97.92 % and least error rate of 2.08 %.

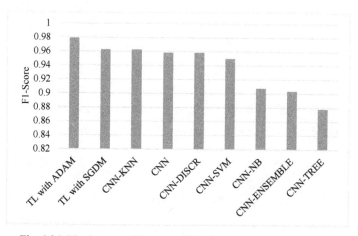

Fig. 4.34 Plot between F1 score and various classification models.

Fig. 4.34 and Fig. 4.35 show the bar chart for F1-score and sensitivity of various models and it is clear that TL with ADAM optimizer has a good F1-score of 0.975 and has a sensitivity of 0.9791.

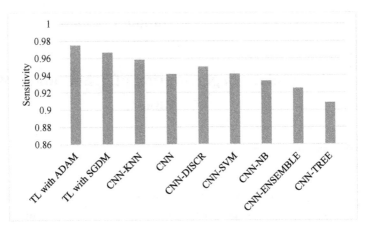

Fig. 4.35 Plot of sensitivity versus various classification models.

4.8 Conclusions

The proposed Transfer learning model is considered for classification of brain tumor MR images as it is much faster and easier when compared to hybrid models. Proposed TL with ADAM optimizer has obtained an accuracy of 97.91 % with an error rate of 2.08 %. Proposed TL with SGDM optimizer and proposed hybrid CNN-KNN model have obtained an accuracy of 96.25 % with an error rate of 3.75 %. An improvement of accuracy 1.71 % is obtained for proposed TL with ADAM optimizer when compared to the proposed TL with SGDM optimizer and hybrid models respectively. An improvement of error rate 80.29 % is obtained for proposed TL with ADAM optimizer when compared to the proposed TL with SGDM optimizer and hybrid models respectively. Hence, the proposed TL model can be used for early detection and classification of brain tumor will increase the chances to treat and cure the patients early and precisely. Extraction of brain tumor sub regions using deep learning models are discussed in the next chapter.

Chapter 5

Sub regions Segmentation of brain tumor of MR images

5.1 Introduction

The application of image processing techniques in the medical field is rapidly increasing in recent years and nowadays, capturing and storing of medical images (Jamroga D et al., 2003) is done digitally. The interpretation of details of medical images is still time consuming. This matter is especially observed in regions with abnormal size and shape which should be identified by radiologists for further studies. Image segmentation (Liu J et al., 2014) is a key task in many image processing and computer vision applications (Patel J and K Doshi, 2014). The purpose of image segmentation is to partition an image into different regions based on a given criteria for further processing. Medical image segmentation (D L Pham et al., 2000) is a key task in many medical applications such as surgery planning, post-surgical assessment, abnormality detection, and so on. The brain image segmentation is a quite complicated, challenging and important task in medical image processing; but image segmentation accuracy is very important to detect enhancing tumors, edema, and necrotic tissues. Early diagnosis of brain tumors plays an important role in improving treatment possibilities and to increase the survival rate of the patients. Manual segmentation (M Prastawa et al., 2004) of the brain tumors for cancer diagnosis from large amount of MRI images generated in clinical data is a difficult and time-consuming task. Most of the manual segmentation techniques fail because of unknown noise, poor image contrast, inhomogeneity and weak boundaries that are usual in medical images. As the medical images mostly contain inherently complex structures and since precise segmentation is necessary for diagnosis, there is a need for automatic brain tumor image segmentation (D Hao et al., 2017). Recently automatic segmentation using deep learning methods became popular, since these methods achieve the state-of-the-art results and can address this problem better than other methods. Deep learning methods also enable efficient processing and objective evaluation of the large amounts of MRI-image data.

This chapter highlights how the brain tumor is extracted from MR image using proposed deep learning model and it's performance is compared with that of clustering algorithms like k-means and fuzzy c-means clustering algorithms. Also brain tumor subregions like Whole Tumor (WT), Tumor Core (TC), and Enhancing Tumor (ET) are extracted using proposed deep learning models. The performance of the proposed models is evaluated in terms of accuracy, error rate, sensitivity, specificity, F1- Score, dice similarity coefficient and Jaccard similarity coefficients. This chapter is organized as follows. Section 5.2 presents overview of existing segmentation methods like Thresholding, Region based, Edge-based, Watershed segmentation, Clustering-based, Artificial Neural Networks (ANN) and Convolutional Neural Network (CNN). Algorithms and architectures of existing clustering methods and proposed deep learning models are discussed in section 5.3. The performance metrics used to evaluate the performance of the models are explained in section 5.4. Section 5.5 and 5.6 deals with experimental results and discussion. Finally, conclusions are given in section 5.7.

5.2   Existing segmentation methods

This section aims to gather and analyze methods used in image segmentation. In general this chapter summarizes suitable image segmentation methods to be used for each type of medical images scan. Segmentations techniques can be divided into the following categories: thresholding-based, region-based, edge-based, Watershed segmentation and clustering-based. Additionally, there are also other methods for image segmentations like ANN and CNN.

5.2.1 Thresholding methods

Thresholding (Gajanayak G et al., 2009) is one of the oldest methods for brain MRI segmentation. This method is very much effective in image binarization, which is an important step in segmentation. Brain tumor in MR image can be defined as regions with pixels having discrete gray level ranges. A particular intensity value known as threshold is defined, which separates the desired regions. Otsu method is a

113

well-established thresholding technique. Otsu method (Otsu N, 1979, Zhang J and J Hu, 2008) is a global thresholding method (Lee S U et al., 1990) in which the pixels in an image are partitioned into two classes (objects and background) at a particular gray level. Total variance, variance within a class, and variance between classes, are calculated. Due to large intensity variation between foreground and background regions, this algorithm will not work perfectly on all brain tumor MR images.

The drawback with this method is finding a threshold level which is a very tough task. If it is failed to select threshold level correctly, the result might be one or all of the following: The segmented region might be smaller or larger than the ground truth, the edges of the segmented region might not be connected, over or under-segmentation of the image (arising of pseudo edges or missing edges).

5.2.2 Region based segmentation

Region growing method (S Gould et al., 2009) extracts regions with similar pixels. Region growing in an image starts with a small element called seed pixel. The adjacent regions having similar properties are combined to form a bigger region. The combination process stops when there are no further regions to merge (J C Tilton et al., 2012). The main criterion for segmentation is the homogeneity of the regions. Gray level, color, texture, shape, etc., are the major criteria for homogeneity. Region splitting and merging (Egenhofer M J and D Wilmsen, 2006) is another type of region based segmentation technique. Here, the image is subdivided into a set of arbitrary regions; these regions are merged or split according to the segmentation algorithm. The set of disjoint regions are coherent to themselves. Advantages of region based segmentation methods are accuracy, simplicity, and choice of multiple criteria. The major disadvantages are extended computational cost and noise sensitivity.

5.2.3 Edge detection

The changes in the intensity of images are used for detecting edges. Edge pixels are those places where image function changes sharply. There are several methods for edge-based segmentation such as Sobel, Prewitt, Roberts, and Canny. Edges normally occur in the boundary between two regions. Edge detection technique (Ziou D and S Tabbone, 1998) makes use of the discontinuities in image values to separate regions. The segmentation algorithm can accurately identify the boundary between these regions. An edge is a region which consists of connected regions of edge pixels. The complexity of edge detection algorithm depends on the ability to localize the edges, noise handling capability, and elimination of false responses. Objects in an image are localized using the edges and the discontinuities will represent the object boundaries. In a sharp image, edges are stronger whereas blurred image consist of weaker edges. The discontinuities in intensity can be calculated using the derivative operator (First order derivative or second order derivative). Merits of this method are simplicity and efficiency in object detection. Demerits of this method are sensitivity to noise, inaccuracy, time consumption, etc.

5.2.4 Watershed segmentation

Watershed segmentation algorithm (Shafarenko L et al., 1997) can be used if the foreground and the background of the image can be identified. Watershed algorithm is also used to capture weak edges. Selection of seed point is the main drawback of this approach. Random selection of seed point may lead to inappropriate results and increases convergence rate. In watershed segmentation an image looks like a surface, where bright pixels are considered as mountain tops and dark pixels are considered as valleys. Some valleys have punctures which are slowly merged into water that will be poured and then it will start to fill the valleys. But if water comes from different punctures, it is not allowed to be mixed. So, the dam is built at contact points which make dams work as boundaries of water and image objects (Deorah S et al., 2006). The steps followed in the watershed segmentation (Srimani P K and Shanthi M, 2013) are,

Step 1: Compute segmentation function,

Step 2: Compute gradient magnitude using derivative operator,

Step 3: Compute foreground markers,

Step 4: Compute background markers,

Step 5: Modify the segmentation function to have minimum values at the foreground and background marker locations.

This method provides very good accuracy as compared to other methods for the detection of brain tumor. The main disadvantage of watershed segmentation is sensitive to intensity variations, due to which over segmentation occurs and this happens mainly when the image is segmented into large number of regions which is not required.

5.2.5 Clustering based algorithm

Clustering is a segmentation technique in which a set of objects in an image are grouped into continuous regions of a multi-dimensional space containing relatively high density of points and low density of points. These regions are separated from each other to form uniform density regions called clusters. Clustering can also be done based on the intensity of the pixels. Hard clustering (Bora D J et al., 2014) is a type of clustering in which data elements belong to only one cluster and the membership value of a region to a particular cluster is exactly 1. In soft clustering, data elements belong to more than one cluster and the membership value of a region to a particular cluster ranges from 0 to 1. The most popular clustering based algorithm are k-means and fuzzy c-means clustering algorithms.

The k-means is an unsupervised clustering algorithm. Initially k number of clusters is selected from the whole image as per a predefined rule. The center of the clusters is chosen randomly during the first iteration. Then the distance (Euclidean) between pixels and center of clusters are calculated. If the distance is near to the center of a particular cluster, then the pixel is moved to that cluster. Otherwise the pixel is moved to the next cluster and so on. The next step is to re-estimate the cluster center. Again each pixel is compared with all centroids and the iteration continues until the center converges.

The advantages of this method are faster computation, reduced complexity, robustness, efficiency, and better result for distinct data sets. The disadvantages are the requirement of prior knowledge (number of clusters) and the inability to handle noisy data. And, if there are 2 highly overlapping data then k-means will not be able to resolve that there are 2 clusters.

Fuzzy C-Means (FCM) is a simple and efficient image clustering algorithm. Here the whole data set is arranged into n distinct groups (clusters). Each data point in the data set is associated with each cluster to a predefined degree. For a particular data point which is closer to the center of a cluster will have high degree of association with that cluster. If the distance between a data point and the cluster center is large, then that data point has less association with the cluster. Initial centers are assumed to mark the location for mean of each cluster. FCM assigns a membership function for each data point in a cluster. Then the cluster centers are randomly moved towards the

116

right. Thus, the membership function gets minimized and represents the distance between any data point to the center of a cluster weighted by the membership function of that point (Dombi J, 1990). The fuzziness of an image and its information content are illustrated by the membership function. FCM provides good segmentation efficiency for overlapped data and data points can belong to more than one cluster. Number of clusters should be assigned manually and lower number of clusters provides better performance.

The FCM algorithm (Chen S and D Zhang, 2004) gives best result for overlapped data set and also gives better result than k-means algorithm. Here, the data point can belong to more than one cluster center. The main drawback of FCM is i) the sum of membership value of a data point in all the clusters must be one but the outlier points has more membership value. So, the algorithm has difficulty in handling outlier points. ii) Due to the influence of all the data members, the cluster centers tend to move towards the center of all the data points. It only considers image intensity thereby producing unsatisfactory results in noisy images. A bunch of algorithms are proposed to make FCM robust against noise and inhomogeneity but it is still not perfect (Balafar M A, 2014, Dave R N, 1991).

5.2.6 Artificial Neural Network

Artificial Neural Networks (ANN) (Sharma M and S Mukharjee, 2012) consist of multiple level of processing elements called nodes which can act like biological neural networks. Elementary computation is performed by each node in an artificial neural network. Highly complex architecture enables the system to produce real time outputs. The system is robust and can perform parallel processing (D Ailing et al., 2016). Propagation function is often a weighted sum, transform or outputs of other neurons in the network. Activation function transforms the network input and sometimes converts old activation function to new activation function. Output function is often an identity function, which transforms activation to output for other neurons. In segmentation scenario, ANN can be used as a clustering method. The major advantages of ANN based segmentation are accuracy, efficiency, robustness, etc. Requirement of training data and high processing time are the major disadvantages of ANN.

117

Neural Network based segmentation (Torbati N et al., 2014) is totally different from conventional segmentation algorithms (Kamdi S and R K Krishna, 2012). In this, an image is firstly mapped into a Neural Network where every Neuron stands for a pixel (Kang, M H and C. P Reynolds, 2009), thus image segmentation problem is converted into energy minimization problem. The neural network can be trained with training sample set in order to determine the connection and weights between nodes. Neural network segmentation includes two important steps: feature extraction and image segmentation based on neural network. Feature extraction is very crucial as it determines input data of neural network (Zhu X and A B Goldberg, 2009), firstly some features are extracted from the images, such that they become suitable for segmentation and then they were the input of the neural network. All of the selected features compose of highly non-linear feature space of cluster boundary. Neural network based segmentation have three basic characteristics: i) High parallel ability and fast computing (W X Kang et al., 2009). ii) Improve the segmentation results when the data deviates from the normal situation (Zhu X and A B Goldberg, 2009). iii) Reduced requirement of expert intervention during the image segmentation process. However, there are some drawbacks of neural networks based segmentation either, such as i) some kind of segmentation information should be known beforehand. ii) Neural network should be trained using learning process beforehand (W X Kang et al. 2009). iii) Period of training may be very long and overtraining should be avoided at the same time.

5.3 Algorithms for brain tumor MR image segmentation

For brain tumor MR image segmentation purpose, clustering and deep learning methods are used in this work. They are k-means clustering, fuzzy c-means clustering, and deep learning models.

5.3.1 k-means algorithm

In k-means algorithm (Wagstaff K et al., 2001, Hooda H et al., 2014, E Abdel-Maksoud, 2015,), initially defines the number of clusters k. Then, the number of k-cluster centroids are taken randomly. The distance between the individual pixels to centers of the individual cluster is measured by means of the Euclidean distance function. A single pixel is compared to all the cluster centroids using the formula for Euclidean distance. Then pixel is moved to the specific cluster having the least distance among all. Then the re-estimation of the centroid is performed. Again each individual pixel is compared to all centroids. This procedure carries on until the cluster centroid converges.

Algorithm steps for K-means:

Step 1: Consider the number of cluster value k.

Step 2: Pick the k cluster centers randomly.

Step 3: Compute cluster's center or mean.

Step 4: Compute the distance between each pixel to each center of the cluster.

Step 5: If the distance is close to the center then move to that particular cluster.

Step 6: Else, move to the subsequent cluster.

Step 7: Re-estimate the center again.

Step 8: Repeat the process until the cluster center does not move.

5.3.2 Fuzzy c-means clustering algorithm

FCM algorithm (Kim T et al., 1988, Szilagyi L, 2003) is one kind of clustering method, which is introduced by Dunn, was enhanced by Bezdek and titivated further by M Matteucci. During segmentation process, only local information is considered in the FCM clustering algorithm. The membership function is permitted to each data point directly related to each cluster center, on the distance between the cluster centroid and data points. The membership function and cluster centers are upgraded after each cycle.

The main FCM objective function is to minimize

$$G(u,v) = \sum_{p=1}^{n} \sum_{q=1}^{k} \left(\mu_{p,q}\right)^{m} \left\|X_p - v_q\right\|^2 \tag{5.1}$$

Where, $\left\|X_p - v_q\right\|^2$ is the Euclidean distance between p^{th} data points and q^{th} cluster centers.

n = Number of data points

v_q = Cluster centroids

m = Fuzziness index m$\epsilon[1,\infty]$

K = Number of cluster centers

119

μ_{pq} = Membership function of data points to cluster centers

d_{pq} = The Euclidean distance between p^{th} data points and q^{th} cluster centers.

Steps for FCM algorithm:

$S = \{s_1, s_2, s_3 ..., s_x\}$ is the data points set and $V_c = \{v_1, v_2, v_3 ..., v_v\}$ is the set of cluster centers.

Step 1: Arbitrarily select k cluster centers.

Step 2: Function of fuzzy membership μ_{pq} is calculated as $\mu_{pq} = \dfrac{1}{\sum_{r=1}^{k}\left(\dfrac{d_{pq}}{d_{pr}}\right)^{\frac{2}{m-1}}}$

Step 3: Calculate fuzzy centers $v_q = \dfrac{\sum_{p=1}^{n}(u_{pq})^m x_p}{\sum_{p=1}^{n}(u_{pq})^m}$

Step 4: Until the G minimum value is accomplished or $\|U_{r+1}-U_r\| < E$, Repeat 2 and 3 steps where,

r = Iteration step

E = Termination criterion is in the range of [0, 1]

$U = (\mu_{pq}) + c$ is the matrix of fuzzy membership.

5.3.3 Proposed deep learning models

Performances of recent deep learning methods, specifically convolutional neural networks (Krizhevsky A et al., 2012), in several object recognition and biological image segmentation challenges increased their popularity among researches. In contrast to traditional classification methods, where hand crafted features are fed into, CNNs automatically learn representative complex features directly from the data itself. Due to this property, research on CNN (Casamitjana A et al., 2016) based brain tumor segmentation mainly focuses on network architecture design rather than image processing to extract features. CNNs take patches extracted from the images as inputs and use trainable convolutional filters and local subsampling to extract a hierarchy of increasingly complex features. Although currently very few number of methods exist to compare with other traditional brain tumor segmentation methods, due to state-of-the-art results obtained by CNN based brain tumor segmentation methods, deep learning models are considered for segmentation task. In addition brain tumor MR image is a 3D data, where, tumor shapes, size, and location can vary greatly from patient to patient. Also tumor boundaries are usually unclear and irregular with discontinuities, because boundaries of the brain tumor are in infiltrative nature. Brain tumor MRI data obtained from clinical scans or synthetic databases are inherently complex. MRI devices and protocols used for acquisition can vary dramatically from scan to scan imposing intensity biases and other variations for each different slice of image in the dataset. The need for several modalities to effectively segment tumor subregions even adds to this complexity. So, situation demands an automatic segmentation model (Isin A et al., 2016, Atkins M S et al., 1998, Cui S et al., 2018) for extracting the brain tumor from brain tumor MR images.

The algorithm and methodology used to solve the problem are described and architecture of the proposed model is also explained in the following sections.

5.3.3.1 Algorithmic description of brain tumor MR image subregions segmentation

Step 1: Assume labels for the data

    No. of patches=4,

    Labels:

        0: others,

        1: necrotic and non-enhancing tumor (NEC+NET),

        2: edema,

        3: original,

        4: enhancing tumor,

        5: complete tumor,

Step 2: Preprocessing

    If label=5   for Complete Tumor (edema)

        Img(img!=0)=1

    If label=1   for NEC+NET

        Img(img!=1)=0

    If label=2   for Tumor Core (NEC+NET+ET)

        Img(img=2)=0

        Img(img!=0)=1

    If label=4   for Enhancing Tumor (ET)

        Img(img!=4)=0

        Img(img=4)=1

Step 3: Normalization of the data with zero mean to avoid zero standard deviation problem.

Step 4: Choose image slice within a range of 60 to 130.

Step 5: Read one subject (patient data).

Step 6: Construct a model for full tumor/enhancing tumor/tumor core.

Step 7: Prepare data for training using T2 modality.

Step 8: Train the model with specified training parameters for maximum number of epoch.

Step 9: Predict the test image for full tumor.

Step 10: To extract enhance tumor and tumor core, prepare training data using T1ce modality and segmented full tumor image. Repeat steps 7 and 8 to get segmented enhancing tumor or tumor core.

5.3.3.2 Methodology of brain tumor MR image subregions segmentation

The deep learning model utilized for brain tumor MRI segmentation is demonstrated based on U-net (Chen W et al., 2018, Feng X and C Meyer, 2017, Norman B et al., 2018) and Visual Geometry Group (VGG16) architectures (Qassim H et al., 2018). Multi modal brain tumor MR images of size of 240 pixels × 240 pixels × 3 channels are applied as input and the database images are in the format of nii, which is usually used for brain imaging data format i.e., Neuroimaging Informatics Technology Initiative. In this methodology, brain tumor subregions like ET, TC and WT are segmented separately. Due to complexity of medical image, applying single modality of the image and using single model are not enough to segment subregions of MRI brain tumor as tumor core is inside of the whole tumor, and enhancing tumor is part of tumor core. To solve the problem, the advantage of whole tumor prediction and calculation of the center point of whole tumor is used, and then the center point is use to crop out the training data for enhancing tumor and Tumor core. The number of cropping images depends on the size of whole tumor and even the overlap part is dropped to do data-augmentation, cropping size is fixed as 64 pixels × 64 pixels. The T1c image is cropped according to center point of the whole tumor prediction. If the patch size is bigger than 64 pixels × 64 pixels, then more than one patch are cropped. Then the 64 pixels × 64 pixels training data is applied to another deep learning model to train and predict. The result of tumor core prediction and enhancing tumor prediction are paste back to original whole tumor prediction according to the center point of it to get combination of all sub regions into one image.

Figure 5.1 presents the proposed approach in a flowchart form. Instead of using all MRI modalities, T2 and Flair data are used for whole tumor segmentation using 23 layers DL model. Only T1c modality for enhancing tumor and tumor core segmentation using 18 layers DL model are used to accelerate training. The whole tumor is mainly obtained by segmenting the T2-weighted images and is utilized to check the edema's extension in T2-weighted FLAIR and discriminate it against ventricles and other necrotic structure. Enhancing tumor and tumor core are both segmented by evaluating the hyper-intensities in T1-weighted contrast enhanced images and patches obtained from full tumor images earlier.

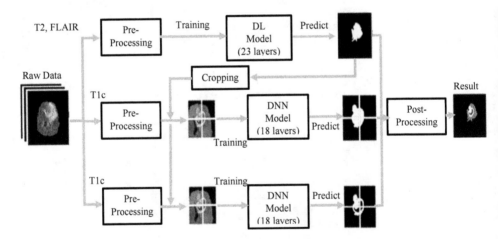

Fig. 5.1 Segmentation of Glioma sub regions using proposed methodology.

5.3.3.3 Deep Learning model architecture

The brain tumor sub regions segmentation process consists of two DL models. Firstly, a 23 layers deep learning model is used to segment full tumor (whole tumor) as shown in the Fig. 5.3. Secondly, this segmentation result is used as input to two 18 layer DL models to segment enhancing tumor and tumor core as shown in the Fig. 5.4. The proposed 18 layers DL model is obtained by removing C4 block from contracting path and E1 block from expanding path.

These proposed DL models are having the following differences from original U-net model

123

i)　　A batch-normalization layer is considered after each convolution layer to stay the gradient levels controlled, speed up convergence and decrease the result of internal covariate shift, so that the network's parameters are not changed rapidly during back propagation,

ii)　　Same padding in convolution layers is used to maintain the feature map size unchanged,

iii)　　Only one final convolution filter is used for binary classification based segmentation, and

iv)　　Two input channels in the input layer used are T2-weighted and FLAIR images for whole tumor segmentation.

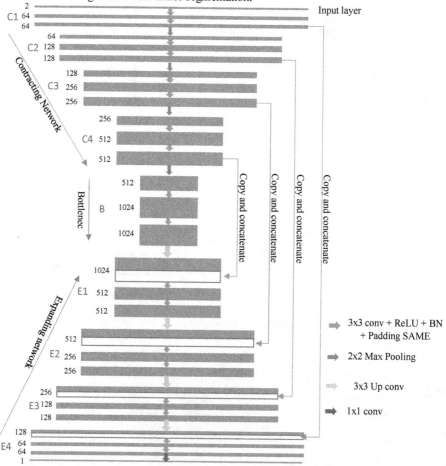

Fig. 5.2 Architecture of proposed deep learning model with auto-encoder structure.

124

Figure 5.2 shows the proposed DL model architecture. The proposed DL model is thought of as an auto-encoder, which consists of contracting path and expanding path. The contracting path tries to learn features of the image, and an expanding path attempts to utilize these features to reconstruct the image with low dimensional data like the ground truth.

The convolution or pooling layers are stacked in the contracting path, whereas in the expanding path up-sampling or transposed convolution layers are incorporated. With the up-sampled output of various phases, high-resolution features from the contracting path are concatenated in order to localize. These are known as skip connections (Milletari F et al., 2016, Drozdzal et al., 2016). The filter size of convolution layers is 3×3 and the same padding is used to keep the output size of convolution layers unchanged are used in each convolution layer and followed by a batch normalization layer. After two convolution layers with batch normalization, a max-pooling of 2×2 with stride of 2 is considered for down-sampling the image size to 1/2. At every down-sampling step the number of feature channels are double. There is an up-sampling of the feature map on each expanding path followed by a 2×2 transposed convolution (up-convolution) halving the number of feature channels, a concatenation with the correspondingly cropped feature map from the contracting path, and two 3×3 convolutional filters. Since each model is based on binary classification based segmentation, the final layer is a 1 pixels $\times$ 1 pixels convolution with one filter, producing binary prediction that 1 is tumor and 0 is non tumor.

Table 5.1 shows the comparison of different layers involved in existing original U-net and the proposed deep learning models architectures. The details of each model are listed in table below where the difference lies in the number of convolutional, ReLU, batch normalization and max pooling layers.

Table 5.1 Layers details of original U-net, proposed DL models with 23 and 18 layers.

Original U-net	Proposed DL Models	
	DL Model (23 layer)	DL Model (18 layer)
Total layers: 47 1 input layer 23 convolutional layers (4- transpose conv) 18 ReLUs 4 maxpooling layers 1 sigmoid (last conv for output layer)	Total layers: 65 1 input layer 23 convolutional layers (4- transpose conv) 18 ReLUs 18 Batch normalization layers 4 maxpooling layers 1 sigmoid (last conv for output layer)	Total layers: 51 1 input layer 18 convolutional layers (3- transpose conv) 14 ReLU 14 Batch normalization layers 3 maxpooling layers 1 sigmoid (last conv for output layer)

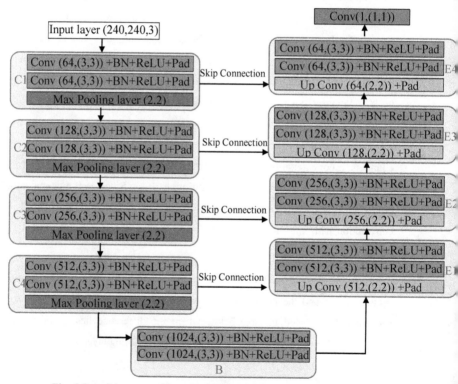

Fig. 5.3 Architecture of proposed 23 layers DL model for Whole Tumor segmentation.

The proposed DL model (23 layers) architecture consists of three parts namely contracting path (C), bottleneck (B), and expanding path (E). The contracting path comprises of 4 blocks C1, C2, C3, and C4. Each block is composed of two 3 × 3 convolution layers, activation function ReLU with batch normalization and one 2 × 2 max-pooling layer. The number of feature maps doubles at each pooling, starting with 64 feature maps for the first block, 128 for the second, and so on. The purpose of this contracting path is to capture the contextual information of the input image. This contextual information is then transferred to expanding path by means of skip connections. Bottleneck is a part of the network that lies between contracting and expanding paths. The bottleneck is built from simply 2 convolutional layers (with batch normalization), with dropout. The expanding path is also composed of 4 blocks E1, E2, E3, and E4. Each of these blocks is composed of Deconvolution layer, Concatenation with the corresponding cropped feature map from the contracting path, two 3 x 3 Convolution layers, and activation function ReLU with batch normalization layer. The purpose of this expanding path is to enable precise localization combined with contextual information from the contracting path. Same padding is used at each layer except at max pooling layer. The final layer is a 1 × 1 convolutional layer with one filter to produce segmented output.

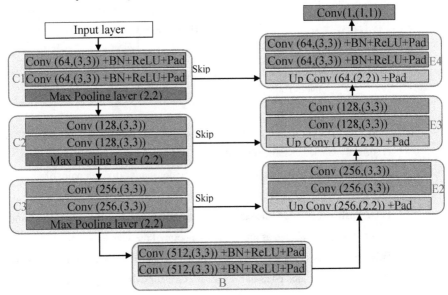

Fig. 5.4 Architecture of proposed 18 layers DL model for Tumor Core and Enhancing Tumor segmentation.

The proposed DL model with 18 layer architecture is similar to proposed DL model with 23 layers which is obtained by removing C4 block from contracting path

127

and E1 block from expanding path. The architecture of proposed 18 layers DL model is shown in the figure 5.4. The proposed model is trained with cropped patches from whole tumor and T1c modality images from original database. Then the trained model is used to segment the tumor core and enhancing tumor.

5.4 Performance evaluation metrics

The performance measures used to evaluate the performance of the proposed methods and model are accuracy, error rate, sensitivity, specificity, F1-measure, dice similarity coefficient, and Jaccard similarity coefficient. Most of the performance metrics are calculated on the bases of the Confusion Matrix as shown in the Table 5.2. Dice similarity coefficient and Jaccard similarity coefficient are also used to measure the surface similarity of the glioma subregions.

Table 5.2 Confusion matrix

Ground truth / Predicted	Tumor (1) (Positive)	Non Tumor (0) (Negative)
Tumor (1)	TP	FP
Non-Tumor (0)	FN	TN

True Positives (TP) are the cases when the tumor (1) data point of ground truth image is correctly labeled as tumor (1) data point of the segmented image.

True Negatives (TN) are the cases when the non-tumor (0) data point of ground truth image is correctly labeled as non-tumor (0) data point of the segmented image.

False Positives (FP) are the cases when the non-tumor (0) data point of ground truth image is wrongly labeled as tumor (1) data point of the segmented image.

False Negatives (FN) are the cases when the tumor (1) data point of ground truth image is correctly labeled as non-tumor (0) data point of the segmented image.

When the person actually not having cancer is classified as cancerous, it is less dangerous than not identifying or capturing a cancerous patient since anyway the cancer cases will be send for further examination and reports. But missing a cancer

128

patient will be a huge mistake as no further examination will be done on them. So that False Negatives should be minimum for a good model or method.

Accuracy is defined as the ratio of number of correctly labeled data points to the total number of data points.

$$\text{Accuracy} = \frac{TP+TN}{TP+TN+FP+FN} \times 100 \qquad (5.2)$$

Accuracy is a good measure when the prediction classes in the data are nearly balanced. That is, every class has same number of samples. For imbalance data, accuracy is not sufficient to evaluate the model, other performance metrics like sensitivity, specificity, F1-score, dice similarity coefficient, and Jaccard similarity coefficient are needed to evaluate the model.

Precision or specificity is defined as the ratio of number of true positives to number of true positives to number of positive calls. It is also called as Positive Predictive Rate (PPR).

$$\text{Specificity} = \frac{TP}{TP+FP} \qquad (5.3)$$

Precision is a measure that tells us what proportion of patients that are diagnosed as having cancer and actually had cancer.

Recall or Sensitivity is defined as probability of a positive test given that the patient has tumor. It is also called as true positive rate.

$$\text{Sensitivity} = \frac{TP}{TP+FN} \qquad (5.4)$$

Recall is a measure that tells us what proportion of patients that actually had cancer was diagnosed by the algorithm as having cancer.

F1 Score is expressed as the accuracy of a test and is interpreted as a weighted average of accuracy and recall.

$$F1 - \text{Score} = \frac{2 \times \text{precision} \times \text{recall}}{\text{precision} + \text{recall}} \qquad (5.4)$$

Error rate is defined as the number of data points which are classified incorrectly to the total number of data points. It can be defined as 1-accuracy.

$$\text{Error rate} = \frac{FP+FN}{TP+TN+FP+FN} \times 100 \qquad (5.5)$$

Dice Similarity Coefficient is a quantity of structural overlap between the predicted image and ground truth image. The lower value of dice score 0 indicates lower spatial overlap between segmented and ground truth images; and the maximum value of dice score 1 indicates higher spatial overlap between segmented and ground truth images.

$$\text{Dice} = \frac{2 \times \text{TP}}{\text{TP+FP+FN}}$$

(5.6)

Jaccard coefficient is another widely used surface overlap measurement, which can be defined as the surface overlap between segmented image and its corresponding ground truth image.

$$\text{Jaccard} = \frac{\text{TP}}{\text{TP+FP+FN}}$$

(5.7)

5.5 Experimental results and discussions

Segmentation of brain tumor MR images is performed using k-means clustering, fuzzy c-means clustering and deep learning model. Each model is compared with other models with performance evaluation metrics like accuracy, error rate, sensitivity, specificity, F1-measure, dice similarity coefficient, and Jaccard similarity coefficient. In addition, brain tumor subregions are extracted using deep learning model and the model is evaluated the model with performance evaluation metrics. Data set considered for segmentation purpose is BraTS 2018 database.

5.5.1 Brain tumor MR image segmentation using k-means clustering algorithm

The implementation of the k-means segmentation method for a brain tumor is performed on the dataset of BraTS2018 database. One image from the dataset is considered to be converted from RGB to gray scale image with size of 240 pixels × 240 pixels and applied to the k-means clustering algorithm. It is an iterative method to update the cluster centroids based on calculating Euclidian distance and stops when the cluster centroids converges.

| 1 | Name of the Patient: Brats18_2013_3_1 |

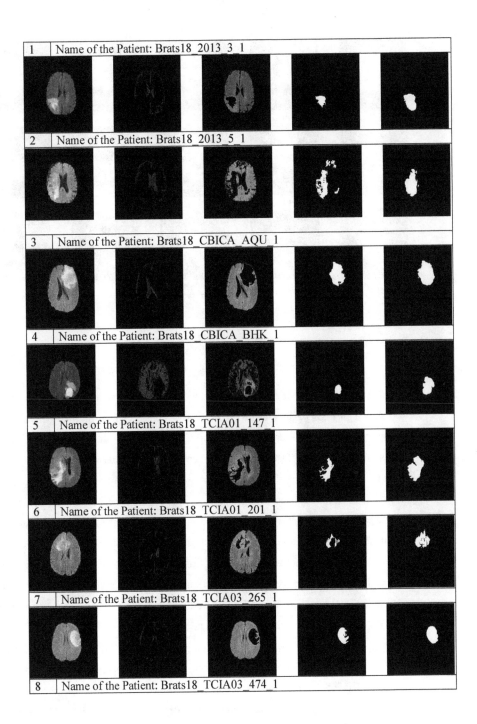

| 2 | Name of the Patient: Brats18_2013_5_1 |

| 3 | Name of the Patient: Brats18_CBICA_AQU_1 |

| 4 | Name of the Patient: Brats18_CBICA_BHK_1 |

| 5 | Name of the Patient: Brats18_TCIA01_147_1 |

| 6 | Name of the Patient: Brats18_TCIA01_201_1 |

| 7 | Name of the Patient: Brats18_TCIA03_265_1 |

| 8 | Name of the Patient: Brats18_TCIA03_474_1 |

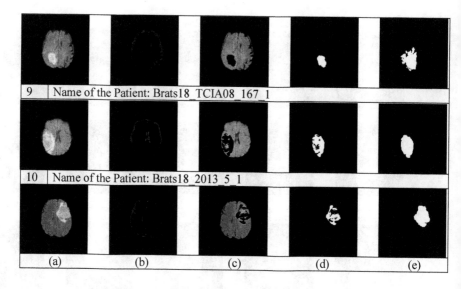

| 9 | Name of the Patient: Brats18_TCIA08_167_1 |
| 10 | Name of the Patient: Brats18_2013_5_1 |

| (a) | (b) | (c) | (d) | (e) |

Fig. 5.5 Brain tumor MRI segmentation using k-means clustering.
a) Original images (FLAIR) b) Clustered image 1 c) Clustered image 2
d) Segmented images e) Ground truth images.

The results of MR image segmentation using k-means clustering algorithms are shown in Fig. 5.5 in a stepwise fashion. It consists of an original MR image, Clustered Image 1, Clustered Image 2, and Clustered image 3 (segmented image) of the brain tumor. Three cluster centroids are chosen and initialized the cluster centroids with initial values of $cc1 = 0.08$, $cc2 = 0.45$, $cc3 = 0.91$ for one incident. Here, these cluster centroids are chosen with normalized pixel values as near to background, brain image part, and tumor part of input image. In each iteration, the Euclidean distance is calculated between data point and each cluster centroids. Then data point (pixel) is moved to the specific cluster having the least distance among all. Then the cluster centroid is re-estimated. Again each individual (data point) pixel is compared to all centroids. This process is stopped when the highest number of iterations are attained or until the cluster centroid converges. The final cluster centers are $ccc1 = 0.1917$, $ccc2 = 0.3300$, $ccc3 = 0.7656$. The fifth image of Fig. 5.5 shows the required segmented image that is obtained by applying area opening operation on the clustered image 3. Table 5.3 shows the performance metrics of confusion matrix for k-means clustering method. For the case Brats18_TCIA08_167_1, the values of TP, FP, TN, and FN are obtained as 2036, 0, 55052, and 512 respectively. Despite the k-means

132

clustering algorithm has good accuracy but it segments more tumor data points or pixels (ground truth image) into non-tumor data points (segmented image). That is FN value in the table shows that more number of cancer cases are missed because the proposed k-means clustering algorithm fails when the data points are belonging to more than one cluster (Fuzziness). To overcome this problem, a fuzzy based clustering algorithm is needed to reduce the false negatives (FN) without compromising the accuracy.

Table 5.3 Confusion matrix of k-means Clustering algorithm.

Name of the Subject	TP	FP	TN	FN
Brats18_2013_3_1	844	0	55835	921
Brats18_2013_5_1	2184	788	54170	458
Brats18_CBICA_AQU_1	2537	0	54491	572
Brats18_CBICA_BHK_1	599	0	55796	1205
Brats18_TCIA01_147_1	1508	0	54749	1343
Brats18_TCIA01_201_1	691	0	55835	1074
Brats18_TCIA03_265_1	1404	0	55753	443
Brats18_TCIA03_474_1	967	0	54924	1709
Brats18_TCIA08_167_1	2036	0	55052	512
Brats18_TCIA08_234_1	1482	0	54825	1293

5.5.2 Brain tumor MR image segmentation using fuzzy c-means clustering

When the data points belong to more than one cluster, the fuzzy c-means clustering algorithm might have better performance than k-means clustering algorithm. An original MR image is converted to gray scale image from RGB image, where Clustered Image is the image obtained when centroids are chosen near to background, brain image, and tumor pixel value of original image.

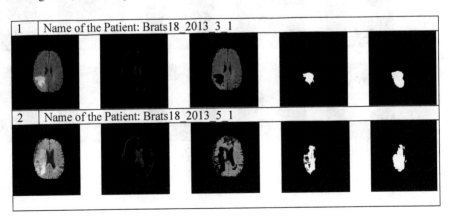

| 1 | Name of the Patient: Brats18_2013_3_1 |
| 2 | Name of the Patient: Brats18_2013_5_1 |

133

3	Name of the Patient: Brats18_CBICA_AQU_1

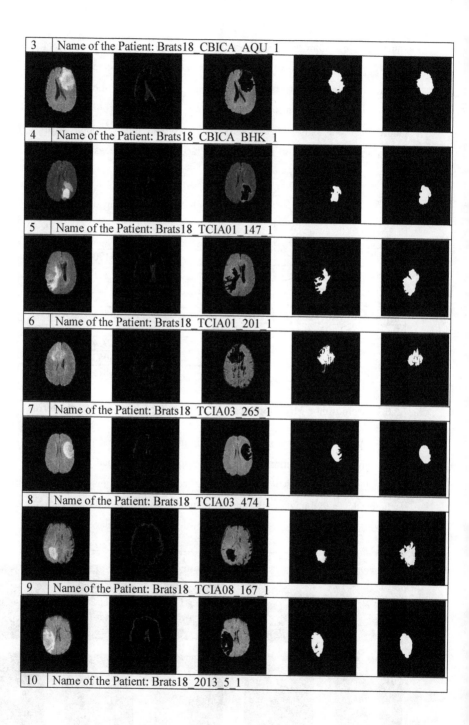

4	Name of the Patient: Brats18_CBICA_BHK_1

5	Name of the Patient: Brats18_TCIA01_147_1

6	Name of the Patient: Brats18_TCIA01_201_1

7	Name of the Patient: Brats18_TCIA03_265_1

8	Name of the Patient: Brats18_TCIA03_474_1

9	Name of the Patient: Brats18_TCIA08_167_1

10	Name of the Patient: Brats18_2013_5_1

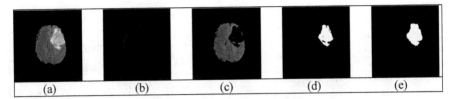

| (a) | (b) | (c) | (d) | (e) |

Fig. 5.6 Brain tumor MR image segmentation using fuzzy c-means clustering algorithm. a) Original images (FLAIR) b) Clustered image 1 c) Clustered image 2 d) Segmented images e) Ground truth images.

The initial fuzzy partition matrix is first generated and then calculated the initial fuzzy cluster center values cc1 = 10.41, cc2 = 84.43, cc3 = 173.32 are taken as an initial cluster centroids. In each iteration, the cluster centers and the membership grade point are updated and the best location for the clusters is obtained by minimizing the objective function. This process is stopped when the highest number of iterations are attained or when the improvement in the objective function between two consecutive iterations is less than specified minimum improvement. The final cluster center values are   ccc1 = 3.8650, ccc2 = 84.5062, ccc3 = 172.5919. The fifth image of Fig. 5.6 shows the required segmented image that is obtained by applying area opening operation on the clustered image 3. The results of MR image segmentation are shown in Fig. 5.6 in a stepwise fashion. The performance measures of confusion matrix for brain tumor segmentation of MRI using fuzzy c-means clustering are recorded in the table 5.4. For the case Brats18_TCIA08_167_1, the values of TP, FP, TN, and FN are obtained as 2334, 7, 55045, and 214 respectively. When this algorithm is compared with k-means clustering algorithm in terms of performance evaluation metrics such as FN and accuracy, this algorithm achieved improved accuracy and reduces FN value drastically. Still there is a scope in improvement to reduce the FN value (missing cancer cases). Since fuzzy c-means and k-means clustering methods require the prior knowledge like number of clusters. Fuzzy c-means offer less segmentation accuracy compared to deep learning models because of the inability to handle noisy data, highly overlapping data. This highly demands an automatic, reproducible, and robust segmentation method to extract the tumor regions from MRI brain tumor. In order to assist the radiologist to take better decision and plan better possible treatment to get cure.

Table 5.4 Confusion matrix of fuzzy c-means clustering.

Name of the Subject	TP	FP	TN	FN
Brats18_2013_3_1	973	0	55835	792
Brats18_2013_5_1	2204	193	54765	438
Brats18_CBICA_AQU_1	2689	2	54489	420
Brats18_CBICA_BHK_1	1234	0	55796	570
Brats18_TCIA01_147_1	1852	0	54749	999
Brats18_TCIA01_201_1	1679	647	55188	86
Brats18_TCIA03_265_1	1453	0	55753	394
Brats18_TCIA03_474_1	1062	0	54924	1614
Brats18_TCIA08_167_1	2334	7	55045	214
Brats18_TCIA08_234_1	2318	0	54825	457

5.5.3 MRI brain tumor segmentation using proposed deep learning models

The proposed deep learning models are trained with BraTS 2018 database. This database consists of 285 glioma patients MRI scan images, among them 210 patients images belongs to High Grade Glioma (HGG III-IV) that is malignant brain tumor images, remaining 75 are Low Grade Glioma (LGG I-II) that is benign brain tumor images. Each patient have four modalities of MRI scan sequences and each modalities again comprising of 155 slices with volumetric images. The four imaging modalities in the BraTS database are described as T1, T1ce, T2, and FLAIR images and all these imaging modalities are available in sagittal view, axial view, and coronal view. The data provided in the BraTS database is preprocessed and ground truths of the training dataset are provided. So that the training dataset in the BraTS database is known as supervised data. The entire work is implemented using the TensorFlow and Keras in python and executed on google colabaratory platform using BraTS 2018 database. The data base is split into two datasets namely training and testing datasets with ratio of 70:30. Here, the imaging modalities of the database are considered from axial view.

The most popular medical image segmentation model U-net and another VGG16 model architectures are considered to make a proposed deep learning model to perform segmentation task. In this study, various subregions of brain tumor like ET, TC, and WT are detected and segmented. A data augmentation is applied to the original dataset to produce more training data virtually. The data augmentation is used here to enhance the efficiency of the network by providing more training data. The data augmentation includes simple transformation like rotation, flipping, shifting, shear operation, brightness, elastic distortion, and zoom. These operations can result in displacement field to images, tumor global shape slightly distorted in horizontal direction and generates more training data.

In preprocessing stage, the data is normalized with zero mean to avoid zero standard deviation problem. Generally, the cross entropy loss evaluates the class label prediction for each pixel vector individually and averages over all pixels. This can be a problem if various classes in the database have unbalanced representation in the image, as training can be dominated by the most prevalent class. Instead of cross entropy loss, a soft dice coefficient loss is used as cost function. It is evaluated for each class separately and then averaged to yield a final score. The stochastic gradient decent momentum is considered as optimizer to minimize the cost function with specified parameters. The adaptive momentum estimator is adopted to estimate the parameters. Here the hyper parameters for training process are considered as learning rate of 0.0001and maximum number of epochs are equals to 60.

To extract whole tumor of MRI brain tumor the proposed DL model of 23 layers is trained with training dataset of 70 percentage of BraTS training dataset with T2-weighted and T2-weigheted FLAIR image modalities of both HGG and LGG cases. The model is evaluated the model on testing dataset of BraTS database with same modality of HGG cases, which was split into 30 percentage of brats training database.

The labels provided in the BraTS database are '1' for NET (non-enhancing tumor) and NCR (necrotic), '2' for ED (Edema), '4' for ET (Enhancing Tumor) or Active Tumor (AT), and 0 for everything else. For each patient, the evaluation has been done on extracting three subregions of MRI brain tumor. The subregions glioma resected as Active Tumor (AT) or ET, WT, and TC. Here whole tumor includes 1, 2 and 4 labels in the labeling of the data. The whole tumor is mainly obtained by segmenting the T2-weighted images and is utilized to check the edema's extension in T2-weighted FLAIR and discriminate it against ventricles and other necrotic structure. Here the whole tumor is considered as segmented image and the performance metrics of confusion matrix are calculated while comparing segmented image with ground truth image.

Table 5.5 Confusion matrix of proposed DL model.

Name of the Subject	TP	FP	TN	FN
Brats18_2013_3_1	1752	45	55790	13
Brats18_2013_5_1	2495	36	54922	147
Brats18_CBICA_AQU_1	3006	86	54405	103
Brats18_CBICA_BHK_1	1780	24	55772	24
Brats18_TCIA01_147_1	2795	56	54693	56
Brats18_TCIA01_201_1	1534	85	55750	231
Brats18_TCIA03_265_1	1830	21	55732	17
Brats18_TCIA03_474_1	2372	68	54856	304
Brats18_TCIA08_167_1	2449	36	55016	99
Brats18_TCIA08_234_1	2759	48	54777	16

The performance measures of confusion matrix for MRI brain tumor segmentation using deep learning are recorded in the Table 5.5. For the case Brats18_TCIA08_167_1, the values of TP, FP, TN, and FN are obtained as 2449, 36, 55016, and 99 respectively. When compared this algorithm with the clustering algorithm in terms of performance evaluation metrics such as FN and accuracy, this algorithm has shown improved accuracy and reduced FN value drastically.

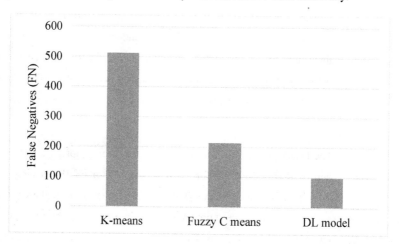

Fig. 5.7 False Negatives (FN) of a patient Brats18_TCIA08_167_1 using proposed DL model.

The Fig. 5.7 shows that the proposed DL model effectively reduced the missing cancer cases by reducing false negative values. The False Negative (FN) values of k-means, fuzzy c-means clustering algorithms and DL model obtained are 512, 214, and 99 respectively.

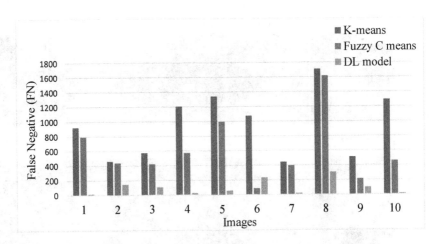

Fig. 5.8 False Negatives (FN) of k-means, fuzzy c-means clustering and proposed DL model.

The Fig. 5.8 clearly shows that the proposed DL model has been reduced the FN values, when compared with other clustering methods it recorded less missing cancer cases for all images.

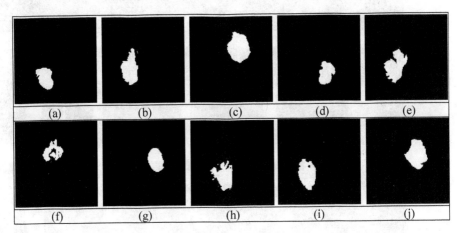

Fig. 5.9 Segmented images of 10 MRI brain tumor patients using proposed DL model.

The whole tumor or segmented image is obtained by DL model of 23 layers trained with T2-weighted and T2-weighted FLAIR image modalities. Randomly 10 patients HGG images are considered for testing and corresponding segmented images are shown in the Fig. 5.9.

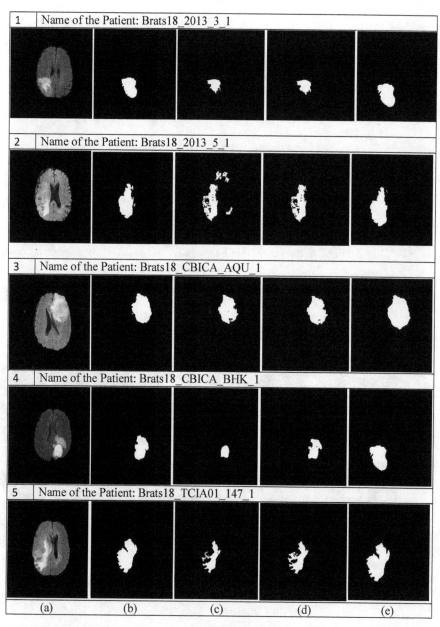

1	Name of the Patient: Brats18_2013_3_1
2	Name of the Patient: Brats18_2013_5_1
3	Name of the Patient: Brats18_CBICA_AQU_1
4	Name of the Patient: Brats18_CBICA_BHK_1
5	Name of the Patient: Brats18_TCIA01_147_1
(a)	(b)	(c)	(d)	(e)

Fig. 5.10 Segmentation results comparison of K-means, fuzzy c-means clustering and Deep Learning models. a) Original image b) Ground truth image c) K-means segmented image d) fuzzy c-means segmented image e) Deep Learning Model segmented image.

The segmentation images of the proposed DL model are compared with other segmentation images of k-means and fuzzy c-means clustering algorithms as shown in the Fig. 5.10. In this figure (a) is an original image, (b) shows the ground truth image of the corresponding patient image, figures c to e show the segmented images of k-means, fuzzy c-means clustering algorithms and DL model.

Here, randomly 10 patients data is chosen for extracting brain tumor and is shown in Table 5.6 to 5.10, and proposed models are evaluated with performance metrics like accuracy, error rate, sensitivity, specificity and considered two more measurements to measure structural overlap between predicted tumor region (in segmented image) to ground truth (in ground truth image).

From Table 5.6 the performance metrics accuracy of 97.9080 %, 99.0104 %, 99.9167 % and error rate of 2.3316 %, 1.7344 %, and 0.1944 % for the patient Brats18_CBICA_BHK_1are obtained using k-means, fuzzy c-means and DL model, respectively. Average accuracy of 98.2087 %, 98.8137 %, 99.7370 % and average error rate of 1.7913 %, 1.1863 %, and 0.2630 % are obtained using k-means, fuzzy c-means and DL model respectively.

Table 5.6 Performance comparison of various segmentation methods in terms of accuracy and error rate.

Name of the Subject	Accuracy			Error-rate		
	k-means	Fuzzy C-means	Proposed DL model	k-means	Fuzzy C-means	Proposed DL model
Brats18_2013_3_1	98.4010	98.6250	**99.8993**	1.5990	1.3750	**0.1007**
Brats18_2013_5_1	97.8368	98.9045	**99.6823**	2.1632	1.0955	**0.3177**
Brats18_CBICA_AQU_1	99.0069	99.2674	**99.6719**	0.9931	0.7326	**0.3281**
Brats18_CBICA_BHK_1	97.9080	99.0104	**99.9167**	2.0920	0.9896	**0.0833**
Brats18_TCIA01_147_1	97.6684	98.2656	**99.8056**	2.3316	1.7344	**0.1944**
Brats18_TCIA01_201_1	98.1354	98.7274	**99.4514**	1.8646	1.2726	**0.5486**
Brats18_TCIA03_265_1	99.2309	99.3160	**99.9340**	0.7691	0.6840	**0.0660**
Brats18_TCIA03_474_1	97.0330	97.1979	**99.3542**	2.9670	2.8021	**0.6458**
Brats18_TCIA08_167_1	99.1111	99.6163	**99.7656**	0.8889	0.3837	**0.2344**
Brats18_TCIA08_234_1	97.7552	99.2066	**99.8889**	2.2448	0.7934	**0.1111**

Table 5.7 Specificity performance evaluation of various segmentation methods.

Name of the Subject	Specificity		
	k-means	Fuzzy C-means	Proposed DL model
Brats18_2013_3_1	1	1	**0.9750**
Brats18_2013_5_1	0.7349	0.9195	**0.9858**
Brats18_CBICA_AQU_1	1	0.9993	**0.9722**
Brats18_CBICA_BHK_1	1	1	**0.9867**
Brats18_TCIA01_147_1	1	1	**0.9804**
Brats18_TCIA01_201_1	1	0.7218	**0.9475**
Brats18_TCIA03_265_1	1	1	**0.9887**
Brats18_TCIA03_474_1	1	1	**0.9721**
Brats18_TCIA08_167_1	1	0.9970	**0.9855**
Brats18_TCIA08_234_1	1	1	**0.9829**

Tables 5.7, 5.8, and 5.9 show the performance of specificity, sensitivity and F1-score for 10 different patients using k-means, fuzzy c-means and proposed DL model respectively. The average values for the proposed DL model in terms of specificity, sensitivity, and F1-score are 0.9776, 0.9572, and 0.9670, respectively.

Table 5.8 Sensitivity performance evaluation of various segmentation methods.

Name of the Subject	Sensitivity		
	k-means	Fuzzy C-means	Proposed DL model
Brats18_2013_3_1	0.4782	0.5513	**0.9926**
Brats18_2013_5_1	0.8266	0.8342	**0.9444**
Brats18_CBICA_AQU_1	0.8160	0.8649	**0.9669**
Brats18_CBICA_BHK_1	0.3320	0.6840	**0.9867**
Brats18_TCIA01_147_1	0.5289	0.6496	**0.9804**
Brats18_TCIA01_201_1	0.3915	0.9513	**0.8691**
Brats18_TCIA03_265_1	0.7602	0.7867	**0.9908**
Brats18_TCIA03_474_1	0.3614	0.3969	**0.8864**
Brats18_TCIA08_167_1	0.7991	0.9160	**0.9611**
Brats18_TCIA08_234_1	0.5341	0.8353	**0.9942**

Table 5.10 shows the performance of dice similarity coefficient and Jaccard similarity coefficients for 10 different patients using k-means, fuzzy c-means and proposed DL model. The average values of k-means, fuzzy c-means, and proposed DL model in terms of dice similarity coefficient are 0.7056, 0.8247, and 0.9670, respectively. The average values of k-means, fuzzy c-means, and proposed DL model in terms of Jaccard similarity coefficients are 0.5638, 0.7155, and 0.9374, respectively.

Table 5.9 F1-Score performance evaluation of various segmentation methods.

Name of the Subject	F1-Score		
	K-means	Fuzzy C-means	Proposed DL model
Brats18_2013_3_1	0.6470	0.7107	**0.9837**
Brats18_2013_5_1	0.7781	0.8748	**0.9646**
Brats18_CBICA_AQU_1	0.8987	0.9272	**0.9695**
Brats18_CBICA_BHK_1	0.4985	0.8124	**0.9867**
Brats18_TCIA01_147_1	0.6919	0.7876	**0.9804**
Brats18_TCIA01_201_1	0.5627	0.8208	**0.9066**
Brats18_TCIA03_265_1	0.8637	0.8806	**0.9897**
Brats18_TCIA03_474_1	0.5309	0.5682	**0.9273**
Brats18_TCIA08_167_1	0.8883	0.9548	**0.9732**
Brats18_TCIA08_234_1	0.6963	0.9103	**0.9885**

Table 5.10 Performance of various segmentation methods in terms of dice and Jaccard similarity coefficients.

Name of the Patient	Dice			Jaccard		
	k-means	Fuzzy C-means	Proposed DL model	k-means	Fuzzy C-means	Proposed DL model
Brats18_2013_3_1	0.6470	0.7107	**0.9837**	0.4782	0.5513	**0.9680**
Brats18_2013_5_1	0.7781	0.8748	**0.9646**	0.6367	0.7774	**0.9317**
Brats18_CBICA_AQU_1	0.8987	0.9272	**0.9695**	0.8160	0.8644	**0.9408**
Brats18_CBICA_BHK_1	0.4985	0.8124	**0.9867**	0.3320	0.6840	**0.9737**
Brats18_TCIA01_147_1	0.6919	0.7876	**0.9804**	0.5289	0.6496	**0.9615**
Brats18_TCIA01_201_1	0.5627	0.8208	**0.9066**	0.3915	0.6961	**0.8292**
Brats18_TCIA03_265_1	0.8637	0.8806	**0.9897**	0.7602	0.7867	**0.9797**
Brats18_TCIA03_474_1	0.5309	0.5682	**0.9273**	0.3614	0.3969	**0.8644**
Brats18_TCIA08_167_1	0.8883	0.9548	**0.9732**	0.7991	0.9135	**0.9478**
Brats18_TCIA08_234_1	0.6963	0.9103	**0.9885**	0.5341	0.8353	**0.9773**

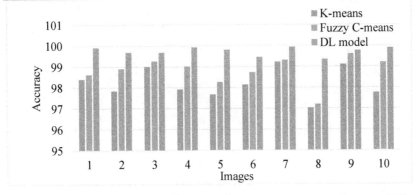

Fig. 5.11 Accuracy comparison of k-means, fuzzy c-means means and proposed DL model for 10 images.

Figure 5.11 indicates the accuracy comparison of 10 images considered and it is observed that the proposed DL model performs better than the existing models k-means and fuzzy c-means model.

Figure 5.12 indicates the error rate comparison of the 10 images taken and it is observed that the proposed DL model has the least error rate than the existing models like k-means and fuzzy c-means model.

Figure 5.13 presents the performance metrics parameters the dice similarity coefficient comparison of the 10 images taken and it is observed that the proposed DL model outperforms in both the parameters than the existing models k-means and fuzzy c-means model.

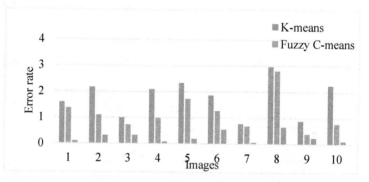

Fig. 5.12 Error rate comparison of k-means, fuzzy c-means and proposed DL model for 10 images.

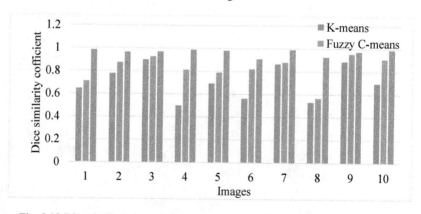

Fig. 5.13 Dice similarity coefficients comparison of k-means, fuzzy c-means and proposed DL model for 10 images.

144

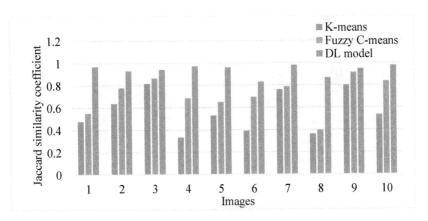

Fig. 5.14 Jaccard similarity coefficients comparison of k-means, fuzzy c-means and proposed DL model for 10 images.

Figure 5.14 presents the performance metrics parameter Jaccard similarity coefficient for the 10 images taken and it is observed that the proposed DL model outperforms than the existing models of k-means and fuzzy c-means model in comparison.

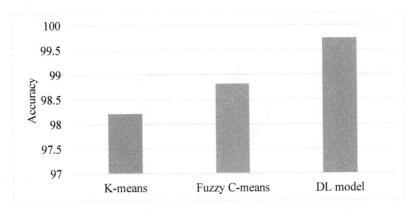

Fig. 5.15 Average accuracy of k-means, fuzzy c-means and proposed DL model.

Figure 5.15 presents the average accuracy in the form of a bar chart for the proposed DL model and compared with the existing models of k-means and fuzzy c-means. It is observed that the proposed DL model nearly achieves 99.62 % accuracy on an average in comparison with the k-means and fuzzy c-means models.

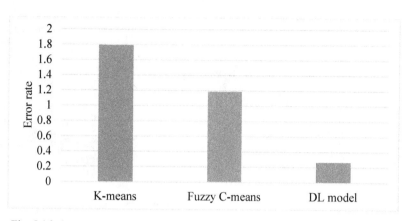

Fig. 5.16 Average error rate of k-means, fuzzy c means and proposed DL model.

Figure 5.16 presents the average error rate in bar chart form for the proposed DL model and compared with the existing models of k-means and fuzzy c-means. It is observed that the proposed DL model nearly has error rate of 0.27 % in comparison with the k-means and fuzzy c-means models.

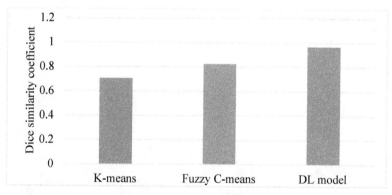

Fig. 5.17 Average dice similarity coefficients of k-means, fuzzy c-means and proposed DL model.

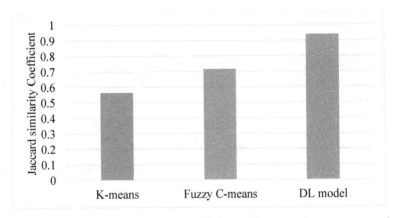

Fig. 5.18 Average Jaccard similarity coefficients of k-means, fuzzy c-means and proposed DL model.

Figure 5.17 and 5.18 present the performance metrics parameters, average values of dice similarity coefficient and Jaccard similarity coefficient of proposed DL model values in comparison with the existing models of k-means and fuzzy c-means and it is observed that the proposed DL model outperforms in both the parameter values when compared with the existing models. The average dice similarity coefficients achieved are 0.98, 0.83, 0.71 and Jaccard similarity coefficients are 0.94, 0.72, and 0.57 for the proposed DL model, fuzzy c-means and k-means clustering, respectively.

5.6 Segmentation of brain tumor subregions in MR image using DL models

The proposed DL model of 18 layers to extracting the subregions like Tumor Core and Enhancing Tumor of brain tumor in MR Image are trained with training dataset of 70 % of BraTS training dataset with T1ce modality and patches of whole tumor both HGG and LGG cases. The model is evaluated on testing dataset of BraTS database with HGG cases, which was split into 30 % of BraTS training database.

The labels provided in the BraTS database are '1' for NET (non-enhancing tumor) and NCR (necrotic), '2' for ED (Edema), '4' for ET (Enhancing Tumor) or Active Tumor (AT), and 0 for everything else. For each patient, the evaluation has been done on extracting three subregions of brain tumor in MR Image. The subregions glioma resected as Active Tumor (AT) or ET, WT, TC. The Enhancing Tumor (ET) is calculated by finding the area of hyper-intensity in the T1Gd or T1c image when contrasted with image T1-weighted, yet additionally when contrasted with healthy white matter in T1c image. The ET is segmented from label 4 in T1ce image modality of Database. The Tumor Core (TC) is segmented by using the combination of labels 1 and 4 in T1c image. And also The TC describes the necrotic regions and the non-enhancing of the tumor. The presence of the NCR and the NET tumor core is regularly hypo-intense in T1c when contrasted with T1. Here whole tumor includes 1, 2, and 4 labels, Tumor Core is combination of 1 and 4 labels, and ET is represented by label 4 only. The WT is complete extension of the tumor and it is primarily segmented from T2 images and cross-check the extension of the edema with T2 weighted FLAIR images and discriminate it against ventricles and other necrotic structure. That is discussed in the section (Section 5.4.3), i.e., brain tumor segmentation in MRI using proposed Deep Learning model (23 layers). A 23-layer deep learning model is used to segment full tumor by training the model with T2 weighted and T2 FLAIR modalities. This segmentation result is used as one of the input and another is T1c images which are applied to train the 18 layers DL model to segment ET and TC separately that as shown in Fig. 5.4.

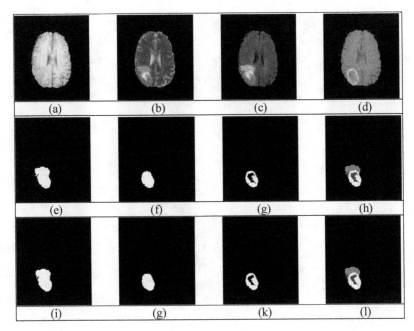

Fig. 5.19 Brain Tumor segmentation of patient name Brats18_2013_3_1 using proposed deep learning models. Images show in first row a to d: T1-weighted image, T2-weighted FLAIR image, T1-constrast image; from second row e to h: Ground truths of whole tumor (WT), tumor core (TC), enhancing tumor (ET), all subregions combination (All); from third row i to l: Prediction of whole tumor (WT), tumor core (TC), enhancing tumor (ET), all subregions combination (All).

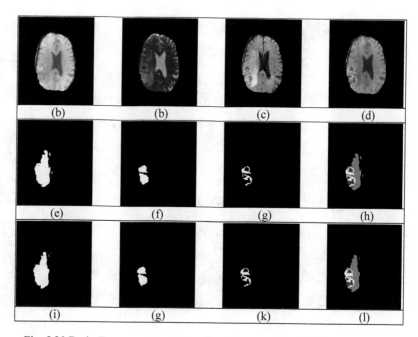

Fig. 5.20 Brain Tumor segmentation of patient name Brats18_2013_5_1 using proposed deep learning models. Images show in first row a to d: T1-weighted image, T2-weighted FLAIR image, T1-constrast image; from second row e to h: Ground truths of whole tumor (WT), tumor core (TC), enhancing tumor (ET), all subregions combination (All); from third row i to l: Prediction of whole tumor (WT), tumor core (TC), enhancing tumor (ET), all subregions combination (All).

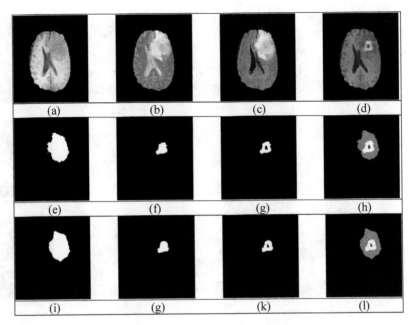

Fig. 5.21 Brain Tumor segmentation of patient name Brats18_CBICA_AQU_1 using proposed deep learning models. Images show in first row a to d: T1-weighted image, T2-weighted FLAIR image, T1-constrast image; from second row e to h: Ground truths of whole tumor (WT), tumor core (TC), enhancing tumor (ET), all subregions combination (All); from third row i to l: Prediction of whole tumor (WT), tumor core (TC), enhancing tumor (ET), all subregions combination (All).

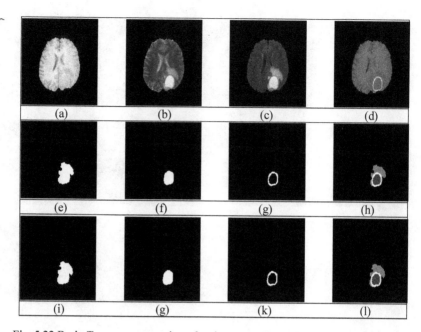

Fig. 5.22 Brain Tumor segmentation of patient name Brats18_CBICA_BHK_1 using proposed deep learning models. Images show in first row a to d: T1-weighted image, T2-weighted FLAIR image, T1-constrast image; from second row e to h: Ground truths of whole tumor (WT), tumor core (TC), enhancing tumor (ET), all subregions combination (All); from third row i to l: Prediction of whole tumor (WT), tumor core (TC), enhancing tumor (ET), all subregions combination (All).

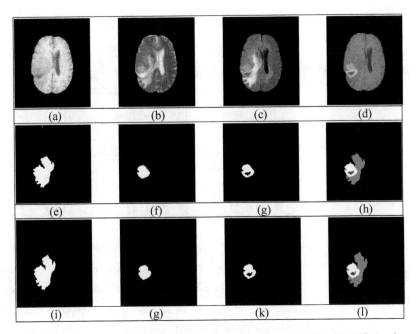

(a)	(b)	(c)	(d)
(e)	(f)	(g)	(h)
(i)	(g)	(k)	(l)

Fig. 5.23 Brain Tumor segmentation of patient name Brats18_TCIA01_147_1 using proposed deep learning models. Images show in first row a to d: T1-weighted image, T2-weighted FLAIR image, T1-constrast image; from second row e to h: Ground truths of whole tumor (WT), tumor core (TC), enhancing tumor (ET), all subregions combination (All); from third row i to l: Prediction of whole tumor (WT), tumor core (TC), enhancing tumor (ET), all subregions combination (All).

Figure 5.19 to 5.23 show randomly considered five patients to extract the subregions of brain tumor in multimodal MR Image using proposed DL models. Images shown in the figure from left to right in first row: T1, T2, FLAIR, and T1ce; from second row: ground truth of whole tumor (Full), ground truth of tumor core (TC), ground truth enhancing tumor (ET), ground truth of all subregions combination (All); from third row: prediction of whole tumor (Full), prediction of tumor core (TC), prediction of enhancing tumor (ET), prediction of all subregions combination (All).

Table 5.11 Performance evaluation metrics accuracy and error rate of tumor core.

Name of the Subject	Accuracy (%)	Error-rate (%)
Brats18_2013_3_1	99.9549	0.0451
Brats18_2013_5_1	99.8507	0.1493
Brats18_CBICA_AQU_1	99.8837	0.1163
Brats18_CBICA_BHK_1	99.9219	0.0781
Brats18_TCIA01_147_1	99.8698	0.1302
Brats18_TCIA01_201_1	99.8646	0.1354
Brats18_TCIA03_265_1	99.9080	0.0920
Brats18_TCIA03_474_1	99.9115	0.0885
Brats18_TCIA08_167_1	99.8507	0.1493
Brats18_TCIA08_234_1	99.8542	0.1458

Table 5.11 and 5.12 show the results of proposed DL model (18 layers) evaluation in terms of performance metrics such as accuracy, error rate, specificity, sensitivity, and F1-score for tumor core subregion. The tumor core is extracted using the proposed DL model (18 layers) with an accuracy of 99.88 %, error rate of 0.11 %, specificity of 0.9798, sensitivity of 0.9004, and F1-score of 0.9291. Considering all the above metrics, it is concluded that the proposed DL model has given outperforming results by reducing false negatives in the prediction phase.

Table 5.12 Performance evaluation metrics specificity, sensitivity, and F1-score of tumor core.

Name of the Subject	Specificity	Sensitivity	F1-Score
Brats18_2013_3_1	0.9913	0.9862	0.9888
Brats18_2013_5_1	0.9704	0.9375	0.9537
Brats18_CBICA_AQU_1	0.9539	0.9498	0.9518
Brats18_CBICA_BHK_1	0.9797	0.9699	0.9748
Brats18_TCIA01_147_1	0.9754	0.9427	0.9588
Brats18_TCIA01_201_1	0.9831	0.4296	0.5979
Brats18_TCIA03_265_1	0.9710	0.9231	0.9464
Brats18_TCIA03_474_1	0.9908	0.9632	0.9768
Brats18_TCIA08_167_1	0.9891	0.9462	0.9672
Brats18_TCIA08_234_1	0.9939	0.9566	0.9749

Table 5.13 and 5.14 show the results of proposed DL model (18 layers) evaluation in terms of performance metrics such as accuracy, error rate, specificity, sensitivity, and F1-score for enhancing tumor subregion. The enhancing tumor is extracted using the

proposed DL model (18 layers) with an accuracy of 99.82 %, error rate of 0.26 %, specificity of 0.9185, sensitivity of 0.8998, and F1-score of 0.8418.

Table 5.13 Performance evaluation metrics accuracy and error rate of enhancing tumor.

Name of the Subject	Accuracy (%)	Error-rate (%)
Brats18_2013_3_1	99.8906	0.1094
Brats18_2013_5_1	99.7396	0.2604
Brats18_CBICA_AQU_1	99.8472	0.1528
Brats18_CBICA_BHK_1	99.8750	0.1250
Brats18_TCIA01_147_1	99.8212	0.1788
Brats18_TCIA01_201_1	99.9479	0.9821
Brats18_TCIA03_265_1	99.9236	0.0764
Brats18_TCIA03_474_1	99.8490	0.1510
Brats18_TCIA08_167_1	99.7153	0.2847
Brats18_TCIA08_234_1	99.6701	0.3299

Table 5.14 Performance evaluation metrics specificity, sensitivity, and F1-score of enhancing tumor.

Name of the Subject	Specificity	Sensitivity	F1-Score
Brats18_2013_3_1	0.9632	0.9703	0.9668
Brats18_2013_5_1	0.8933	0.8799	0.8865
Brats18_CBICA_AQU_1	0.9458	0.9202	0.9328
Brats18_CBICA_BHK_1	0.9256	0.9176	0.9216
Brats18_TCIA01_147_1	0.9553	0.9230	0.9389
Brats18_TCIA01_201_1	0.6548	0.7857	0.0521
Brats18_TCIA03_265_1	0.9955	0.9127	0.9523
Brats18_TCIA03_474_1	0.9657	0.9231	0.9439
Brats18_TCIA08_167_1	0.9757	0.8831	0.9271
Brats18_TCIA08_234_1	0.9104	0.8830	0.8965

Here, randomly 10 patients data is chosen for extracting the subregions like ET, TC, and WT as shown in the figures and evaluated the proposed models and methodology with performance metrics dice similarity coefficient and Jaccard similarity coefficient. For patient Brats18_TCIA01_147_1, Fig. 5.23 shows precise subregions segmentation of brain tumor in multimodal MR Image using the proposed methodology as shown in Fig. 5.1. TC, ET, and WT, are accurately extracted with dice similarity coefficient of 0.9588, 0.9389, and 0.9804 respectively and Jaccard similarity coefficient of 0.9208, 0.8848, and 0.9615 respectively. This result assists the radiologists and doctors to detect the exact size, shape (structural), location of the subregions of brain tumor.

Table 5.15 Comparison of dice similarity coefficient for ET, TC, and WT.

Name of the Subject	Dice		
	Tumor Core	Enhancing Tumor	Whole Tumor
Brats18_2013_3_1	0.9888	0.9668	0.9837
Brats18_2013_5_1	0.9537	0.8865	0.9646
Brats18_CBICA_AQU_1	0.9518	0.9328	0.9695
Brats18_CBICA_BHK_1	0.9748	0.9216	0.9867
Brats18_TCIA01_147_1	0.9588	0.9389	0.9804
Brats18_TCIA01_201_1	0.5979	0.7857	0.9066
Brats18_TCIA03_265_1	0.9464	0.9523	0.9897
Brats18_TCIA03_474_1	0.9768	0.9439	0.9273
Brats18_TCIA08_167_1	0.9672	0.9271	0.9732
Brats18_TCIA08_234_1	0.9749	0.8965	0.9885

From Table 5.15 subregions of brain tumor in MR image are calculated in terms of structural overlap similarity dice coefficient. It shows that how much of the extracted subregion is structurally similar to the ground truth subregion of brain tumor in MR image. The results show that the extracted sub regions like ET, TC, and WT are very close to average dice scores of ground truths with 0.91521, 0.92811, and 0.96702.

Table 5.16 Comparison of jaccard similarity coefficient for ET, TC, and WT.

Name of the Subject	Jaccard		
	Tumor Core	Enhancing Tumor	Whole Tumor
Brats18_2013_3_1	0.9778	0.9356	0.9680
Brats18_2013_5_1	0.9114	0.7962	0.9317
Brats18_CBICA_AQU_1	0.9081	0.8741	0.9408
Brats18_CBICA_BHK_1	0.9508	0.8545	0.9737
Brats18_TCIA01_147_1	0.9208	0.8848	0.9615
Brats18_TCIA01_201_1	0.4265	0.6471	0.8292
Brats18_TCIA03_265_1	0.8983	0.9089	0.9797
Brats18_TCIA03_474_1	0.9546	0.8938	0.8644
Brats18_TCIA08_167_1	0.9364	0.8641	0.9478
Brats18_TCIA08_234_1	0.9510	0.8124	0.9773

From Table 5.16 subregions of brain tumor in MR image are calculated in terms of another structural overlap similarity jaccard coefficient. It shows that how much of the extracted subregion is structurally similar to the ground truth subregion of brain tumor in MR image. The results show that the extracted subregions like ET, TC, and WT are very close to ground truths with average Jaccard scores of 0.84715, 0.88357, and 0.93741.

Table 5.17 Comparison of dice similarity coefficient of deep learning models with other models.

Method	Dice		
	Tumor Core	Enhancing Tumor	Whole Tumor
Stawiaski (NVDLMED) [16]	0.85	0.79	0.91
Xue Feng et al (MIC-KFZ) [17]	0.84	0.79	0.91
Richard McKinley et al (SCAN) [18]	0.80	0.70	0.88
Pereira16 [8]	0.65	0.75	0.79
Havaei16 [11]	0.58	0.69	0.79
Kamnitsas17 [12]	0.76	0.73	0.90
Hao Dong et al. [1]	0.86	0.65	0.86
Proposed model (DL Model)	0.92	0.91	0.96

From Table 5.17, the first three models are trained on BraTS 2018 database. These models stood in first three places in BraTS 2018 challenge and the obtained dice scores are tabulated for brain tumor subregions segmentation. In BraTs 2017 challenge, Pereira16, Havaei16, Kamnitsas17, and Hao Dong et al stood in the first three positions and their dice scores obtained are tabulated in the Table 5.17.

The proposed DL models have been evaluated with randomly selected 10 untrained HGG cases of BraTS 2018 training dataset and already defined testing dataset, and the average values are recorded in Table 5.17. The results show that the extracted sub regions, ET, TC, and WT are very close to their respective ground truths with average dice scores and jaccard scores of 0.91, 0.92, and 0.96 and 0.84, 0.88, and 0.93 respectively.

Figure 5.24, 5.25, and 5.26 present the tumor core, enhancing tumor and whole tumor versus dice similarity coefficient for the different models considered for comparison in this thesis.

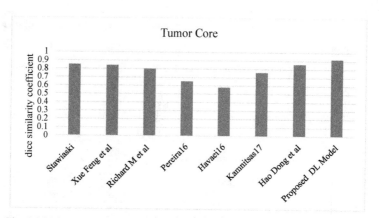

Fig. 5.24 Plot of tumor core versus various models in terms of dice similarity coefficient.

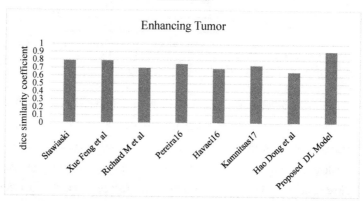

Fig.5.25 Plot of enhancing tumor versus various models in terms of dice similarity coefficient.

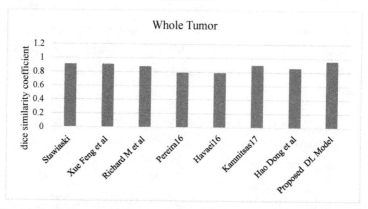

Fig. 5.26 Plot of whole tumor versus various models in terms of dice similarity coefficient.

5.7 Conclusions

Segmentation of brain tumor glioma subregions is performed using two proposed DL models in this chapter. With 23 layers deep learning model, an Average accuracy of 98.20 %, 98.81 %, 99.74 % and average error rate of 1.79 %, 1.19 %, and 0.26 % are obtained for whole tumor extraction using k-means, fuzzy c-means and proposed DL model respectively. The extracted whole tumor is further used with an 18 layers DL model and T1c image to obtain the subregions ET and TC. The performance of the proposed models are evaluated on parameters like accuracy, error rate, sensitivity, specificity, F1-measure, dice similarity coefficient, and Jaccard similarity coefficient. An average dice coefficients of 0.96702, 0.9281, 0.9152 and Jaccard coefficients of 0.9374, 0.8835, 0.8471 and an accuracy of 99.82 %, 99.88 %, and 99.73 %, are attained for ET, TC, and WT, respectively. The overall conclusions are discussed in the next chapter.

Chapter 6

Conclusions and Future Scope of the Work

Tumors can be benign (Noncancerous) or malignant (Cancerous) which have different features and can be identified through brain tumor MR imaging. Different standards for grading of tumors are given by World Health Organization (WHO) and a grade indicates the severity of the tumor. Doctors may identify the type of tumor based on the observations in the brain tumor images and accordingly plan for effective treatment. The BraTS 2018 database is used for training and evaluation of model performance. In this database, the structural information (subregions) and their labels of brain tumor MR images for segmentation task are discussed. (Ch.2).

The performance of PSNR for Gaussian noise corrupted image is improved to 14.24 % in the proposed DeepCNN model for a noise level of 5 and an improvement of 7.66 % is achieved with speckle noise addition. For a Gaussian noise with known noise level of 15, the proposed DeepCNN model shows an improvement of PSNR in dB of 8.39 %. The proposed DeepCNN model appears to be better for reducing noise when image gets corrupted by either speckle or Gaussian noise with known or unknown noise levels. In addition, the proposed DeepCNN preserves the structural information of the image by observing the SSIM values from the results. (Ch.3).

The proposed Transfer Learning model considered for classification of brain tumor MR images is much faster and easier when compared to hybrid models. The proposed TL with ADAM optimizer has obtained an accuracy of 97.91 % with an error rate of 2.08 %. Proposed TL with SGDM optimizer and proposed hybrid CNN-KNN model achieved same accuracy of 96.25 % with an error rate of 3.75 %. An improvement of 1.71 % in accuracy is obtained for proposed TL with ADAM optimizer when compared to the proposed TL with SGDM optimizer and hybrid models respectively. An improvement of error rate of 80.29 % is achieved considering proposed TL with ADAM optimizer when compared to the proposed TL with SGDM optimizer and hybrid models respectively. Hence, the proposed TL model can be used for early detection and classification of brain tumor which will increase the chances of treatment and curing the patients effectively. (Ch.4)

Segmentation of brain tumor glioma subregions is performed using two proposed DL models. With the 23 layer deep learning model, an average accuracy of 98.20 %, 98.81 %, 99.74 % and average error rate of 1.79 %, 1.19 %, and 0.26 % are achieved for whole tumor extraction using K-means, Fuzzy C-means and DL model respectively. The extracted whole tumor is further used with an 18 layer DL model and T1c image to obtain the subregions ET and TC. The performance of the proposed models are evaluated on parameters like accuracy, error rate, sensitivity, specificity, F1-measure, dice similarity coefficient, and Jaccard similarity coefficient. An average dice coefficients of 0.96702, 0.9281, 0.9152, and Jaccard coefficients of 0.9374, 0.8835, 0.8471 and an accuracy of 99.82 %, 99.88 %, and 99.73 %, are attained for ET, TC, and WT respectively. (Ch.5).

Future Scope

As a result of the investigations carried out in this thesis, the following aspects will provide the scope for extending this work to the next level. To detect various types of tumor in all the parts of human body like liver, breast, lungs, etc. and also the work can be extended to find the patient survival rate; the work can also be useful for disease detection in plant leaves and cropping, applying data augmentation transformation to model enlarges the database in order to avoid over-fitting problems advanced pretrained CNN model can be used for faster implementation and better accuracy can be achieved through further tuning of hyper parameters and also develop new network architectures with custom loss function to improve the performance.

References

1. Abdel-Maksoud, Eman, Mohammed Elmogy, and Rashid Al-Awadi. "Brain tumor segmentation based on a hybrid clustering technique." Egyptian Informatics Journal 16, no. 1 (2015): 71-81.

2. Abiwinanda, Nyoman, Muhammad Hanif, S. Tafwida Hesaputra, Astri Handayani, and Tati Rajab Mengko. "Brain tumor classification using convolutional neural network." In World Congress on Medical Physics and Biomedical Engineering 2018, pp. 183-189. Springer, Singapore, 2019.

3. Ahmed, Kaoutar B., Lawrence O. Hall, Dmitry B. Goldgof, Renhao Liu, and Robert A. Gatenby. "Fine-tuning convolutional deep features for MRI based brain tumor classification." In Medical Imaging 2017: Computer-Aided Diagnosis, vol. 10134, p. 101342E. International Society for Optics and Photonics, 2017.

4. Ahmed, Mohamed N., Sameh M. Yamany, Nevin Mohamed, Aly A. Farag, and Thomas Moriarty. "A modified fuzzy c-means algorithm for bias field estimation and segmentation of MRI data." IEEE transactions on medical imaging 21, no. 3 (2002): 193-199.

5. Ajala Funmilola, A., O. A. Oke, T. O. Adedeji, O. M. Alade, and E. A. Adewusi. "Fuzzy kc-means clustering algorithm for medical image segmentation." Journal of Information Engineering and Applications, ISSN 22245782 (2012): 2225-0506.

6. Ali, Jafar MH, and Aboul Ella Hassanien. "PCNN for detection of masses in digital mammogram." Neural Network World 16, no. 2 (2006): 129.

7. Amin, Javeria, Muhammad Sharif, Mussarat Yasmin, and Steven Lawrence Fernandes. "Big data analysis for brain tumor detection: Deep convolutional neural networks." Future Generation Computer Systems 87 (2018): 290-297.

8. Anitha, V., and S. Murugavalli. "Brain tumour classification using two-tier classifier with adaptive segmentation technique." IET computer vision 10, no. 1 (2016): 9-17.

9. Atkins, M. Stella, and Blair T. Mackiewich. "Fully automatic segmentation of the brain in MRI." IEEE transactions on medical imaging 17, no. 1 (1998): 98-107.

10. Aubert, Gilles, and Jean-Francois Aujol. "A variational approach to removing multiplicative noise." SIAM journal on applied mathematics 68, no. 4 (2008): 925-946.

11. Bach Cuadra, M., et al. "Atlas-based segmentation of pathological MR brain images using a model of lesion growth." IEEE trans. on medical imaging 23, no. ARTICLE (2004): 1301-1314.

12. Bakas, Spyridon, Hamed Akbari, Aristeidis Sotiras, Michel Bilello, Martin Rozycki, Justin S. Kirby, John B. Freymann, Keyvan Farahani, and Christos Davatzikos. "Advancing the cancer genome atlas glioma MRI collections with expert segmentation labels and radiomic features." Scientific data 4 (2017a): 170117.

13. Bakas, Spyridon, Hamed Akbari, Aristeidis Sotiras, Michel Bilello, Martin Rozycki, Justin Kirby, John Freymann, Keyvan Farahani, and Christos Davatzikos. "Segmentation labels and radiomic features for the pre-operative scans of the TCGA-LGG collection." The Cancer Imaging Archive 286 (2017b).

14. Balafar, M. A. "Fuzzy C-mean based brain MRI segmentation algorithms." Artificial intelligence review 41, no. 3 (2014): 441-449.

15. Banerjee, Imon, Alexis Crawley, Mythili Bhethanabotla, Heike E. Daldrup-Link, and Daniel L. Rubin. "Transfer learning on fused multiparametric MR images for classifying histopathological subtypes of rhabdomyosarcoma" Computerized Medical Imaging and Graphics 65 (2018): 167-175.

16. Barakbah, Ali Ridho, and Yasushi Kiyoki. "A pillar algorithm for k-means optimization by distance maximization for initial centroid designation." In 2009 IEEE Symposium on Computational Intelligence and Data Mining, pp. 61-68. IEEE, 2009.

17. Bergsneider, Marvin, David A. Hovda, Ehud Shalmon, Daniel F. Kelly, Paul M. Vespa, Neil A. Martin, Michael E. Phelps et al. "Cerebral hyperglycolysis following severe traumatic brain injury in humans: a positron emission tomography study." Journal of neurosurgery 86, no. 2 (1997): 241-251.

18. Bilaniuk, Larissa T., Robert A. Zimmerman, P. Littman, E. Gallo, L. B. Rorke, D. A. Bruce, and L. Schut. "Computed tomography of brain stem gliomas in children." Radiology 134, no. 1 (1980): 89-95.

19. Bin-Habtoor, Abdulaziz Saleh Yeslem, and Salem Saleh Al-amri. "Removal speckle noise from medical image using image processing techniques." International Journal of Computer Science and Information Technologies 7, no. 1 (2016): 375-377.

20. Bin-Habtoor, Abdulaziz Saleh Yeslem, and Salem Saleh Al-amri. "Removal speckle noise from medical image using image processing techniques." International Journal of Computer Science and Information Technologies 7, no. 1 (2016): 375-377.

21. Bishop, C. M. Pattern Recognition and Machine Learning. Springer, New York, NY, 2006.

22. Bora, Dibya Jyoti, Dr Gupta, and Anil Kumar. "A comparative study between fuzzy clustering algorithm and hard clustering algorithm." arXiv preprint arXiv:1404.6059 (2014).

23. Buades, A, Bartomeu C, and Jean-Michel M. "A review of image de-noising algorithms, with a new one." Multiscale Modeling & Simulation 4, no. 2 (2005b): 490-530.

24. Buades, B. Coll, and J.-M. Morel, "A non-local algorithm for image de-noising," in IEEE Conference on Computer Vision and Pattern Recognition, vol. 2, 2005a, pp. 60–65.

25. Buehring, Gertrude Case, and Robert R. Williams. "Growth rates of normal and abnormal human mammary epithelia in cell culture." Cancer research 36, no. 10 (1976): 3742-3747.

26. Burger, Harold C., Christian J. Schuler, and Stefan Harmeling. "Image denoising: Can plain neural networks compete with BM3D?." In Computer Vision and Pattern Recognition (CVPR), 2012 IEEE Conf. on, pp. 2392-2399. IEEE, 2012.

27. Casamitjana, Adria, Santi Puch, Asier Aduriz, and Verónica Vilaplana. "3D Convolutional Neural Networks for Brain Tumor Segmentation: a comparison of multi-resolution architectures." In International Workshop on Brainlesion: Glioma, Multiple Sclerosis, Stroke and Traumatic Brain Injuries, pp. 150-161. Springer, Cham, 2016.

28. Chang, S. Grace, Bin Yu, and Martin Vetterli. "Adaptive wavelet thresholding for image denoising and compression." IEEE transactions on image processing 9, no. 9 (2000): 1532-1546.

29. Chen, Songcan, and Daoqiang Zhang. "Robust image segmentation using FCM with spatial constraints based on new kernel-induced distance measure." IEEE Transactions on Systems, Man, and Cybernetics, Part B (Cybernetics) 34, no. 4 (2004): 1907-1916.

30. Chen, Wei, Boqiang Liu, Suting Peng, Jiawei Sun, and Xu Qiao. "S3D-UNet: separable 3D U-Net for brain tumor segmentation." In International MICCAI Brainlesion Workshop, pp. 358-368. Springer, Cham, 2018.

31. Cihangiroglu, Mutlu, Ruth G. Ramsey, and George J. Dohrmann. "Brain injury: analysis of imaging modalities." Neurological research 24, no. 1 (2002): 7-18.

32. Cintra, R. J., L. C. Rêgo, G. M. Cordeiro, and A. D. C. Nascimento. "Beta generalized normal distribution with an application for SAR image processing." Statistics 48, no. 2 (2014): 279-294.

33. Cui, Shaoguo, Lei Mao, Jingfeng Jiang, Chang Liu, and Shuyu Xiong. "Automatic semantic segmentation of brain gliomas from MRI images using a deep cascaded neural network." Journal of healthcare engineering 2018 (2018).

34. D. E. Rumelhart, J. L. McClelland, and C. PDP Research Group, eds., Parallel Distributed Processing: Explorations in the Microstructure of Cognition, Vol.1: Foundations. Cambridge, MA, USA: MIT Press, 1986.

35. D. P. Kingma and J. Ba, "Adam: A method for stochastic optimization," CoRR, vol. abs/1412.6980, 2014.

36. Dave, Rajesh N. "Characterization and detection of noise in clustering." Pattern Recognition Letters 12, no. 11 (1991): 657-664.

37. De, Ailing, Yuan Zhang, and Chengan Guo. "A parallel adaptive segmentation method based on SOM and GPU with application to MRI image processing." Neurocomputing 198 (2016): 180-189.

38. Deorah, Sundeep, Charles F. Lynch, Zita A. Sibenaller, and Timothy C. Ryken. "Trends in brain cancer incidence and survival in the United States: Surveillance, Epidemiology, and End Results Program, 1973 to 2001." Neurosurgical focus 20, no. 4 (2006): E1.

39. Dombi, J. "Membership function as an evaluation." Fuzzy sets and systems 35, no. 1 (1990): 1-21.

40. Dong, Hao, Guang Yang, Fangde Liu, Yuanhan Mo, and Yike Guo. "Automatic brain tumor detection and segmentation using u-net based fully

convolutional networks." In annual conference on medical image understanding and analysis, pp. 506-517. Springer, Cham, 2017.

41.   Dou, Qi, Hao Chen, Lequan Yu, Lei Zhao, Jing Qin, Defeng Wang, Vincent CT Mok, Lin Shi, and Pheng-Ann Heng. "Automatic detection of cerebral microbleeds from MR images via 3D convolutional neural networks." IEEE transactions on medical imaging 35, no. 5 (2016): 1182-1195.

42.   Drevelegas, Antonios, and Nickolas Papanikolaou. "Imaging modalities in brain tumors." In Imaging of brain tumors with histological correlations, pp. 13-33. Springer, Berlin, Heidelberg, 2011.

43.   Drozdzal, et al. "The importance of skip connections in biomedical image segmentation." In Deep Learning and Data Labeling for Medical Appls., pp. 179-187. Springer, Cham, 2016.

44.   Egenhofer, Max J., and Dominik Wilmsen. "Changes in topological relations when splitting and merging regions." In Progress in Spatial Data Handling, pp. 339-352. Springer, Berlin, Heidelberg, 2006.

45.   F. Isensee, P. Kickingereder, W. Wick, M. Bendszus, and K. H. Maier-Hein, "Brain tumor segmentation and radiomics survival prediction: Contribution to the brats 2017 challenge," in Multimodal Brain Tumor Segmentation Benchmark, Brain-lesion Workshop, MICCAI 2017, 09/2017 2017.

46.   F. Rosenblatt, "The perceptron: A probabilistic model for information storage and organization in the brain," Psychological Review, vol. 65, no. 6, pp. 386–408, 1958.

47.   Feng, Xue, and Craig Meyer. "Patch-based 3D U-Net for brain tumor segmentation." In International Conference on Medical Image Computing and Computer-Assisted Intervention (MICCAI). 2017.

48.   Feng, Xue, et al. "Brain tumor segmentation using an ensemble of 3D u-nets and overall survival prediction using radiomic features." In Int. MICCAI Brainlesion Workshop, pp. 279-288. Springer, Cham, 2018.

49.   Gajanayake, G. M. N. R., Roshan Dharshana Yapa, and B. Hewawithana. "Comparison of standard image segmentation methods for segmentation of brain tumors from 2D MR images." In 2009 International Conference on Industrial and Information Systems (ICIIS), pp. 301-305. IEEE, 2009.

50.   Giesexs, Alf, and Manfred Westphal. "Glioma invasion in the central nervous system." Neurosurgery 39, no. 2 (1996): 235-252.

51. Gonzales, Rafael C., and Richard E. Woods. "Digital image processing." (2002).

52. Gould, Stephen, Tianshi Gao, and Daphne Koller. "Region-based segmentation and object detection." In Advances in neural information processing systems, pp. 655-663. 2009.

53. H. Robbins and S. Monro, "A stochastic approximation method," Ann. Math. Statist., vol. 22, pp. 400–407, 09 1951.

54. Hasan, Mahmud, and Mahmoud R. El-Sakka. "Improved BM3D image denoising using SSIM-optimized Wiener filter." EURASIP journal on image and video processing 2018, no. 1 (2018): 25.

55. Havaei, M, et al. "Brain tumor segmentation with deep neural networks." Medical image analysis 35 (2017): 18-31.

56. Holly, Thomas A., Brian G. Abbott, Mouaz Al-Mallah, Dennis A. Calnon, Mylan C. Cohen, Frank P. DiFilippo, Edward P. Ficaro et al. "Single photon-emission computed tomography." Journal of nuclear cardiology 17, no. 5 (2010): 941-973.

57. Hooda, Heena, Om Prakash Verma, and Tripti Singhal. "Brain tumor segmentation: A performance analysis using K-Means, Fuzzy C-Means and Region growing algorithm." In 2014 IEEE International Conference on Advanced Communications, Control and Computing Technologies, pp. 1621-1626. IEEE, 2014.

58. Hu, Kai, et al. "Brain Tumor Segmentation Using Multi-Cascaded Convolutional Neural Networks and Conditional Random Field." IEEE Access 7 (2019): 92615-92629.

59. Ioffe, Sergey, and Christian Szegedy. "Batch normalization: Accelerating deep network training by reducing internal covariate shift." arXiv preprint arXiv:1502.03167 (2015).

60. Iqbal, Sajid, et al. "Brain tumor segmentation in multi-spectral MRI using convolutional neural networks (CNN)." Microscopy research and technique 81, no. 4 (2018): 419-427.

61. Isensee, Fabian, et al. "No new-net." In International MICCAI Brainlesion Workshop, pp. 234-244. Springer, Cham, 2018.

62. Işın, Ali, Cem Direkoğlu, and Melike Şah. "Review of MRI-based brain tumor image segmentation using deep learning methods." Procedia Computer Science 102 (2016): 317-324.

63. Işın, Ali, et al. "Review of MRI-based brain tumor image segmentation using deep learning methods." Procedia Comput. Sci. 102 (2016): 317-324.

64. Islam, Atiq, Syed MS Reza, and Khan M. Iftekharuddin. "Multifractal texture estimation for detection and segmentation of brain tumors." IEEE transactions on biomedical engineering 60, no. 11 (2013): 3204-3215.

65. J. Duchi, E. Hazan, and Y. Singer, "Adaptive subgradient methods for online learning and stochastic optimization," Tech. Rep. UCB/EECS-2010-24, EECS Department, University of California, Berkeley, Mar 2010.

66. J. Kiefer and J. Wolfowitz, "Stochastic estimation of the maximum of a regression function," Ann. Math. Statist., vol. 23, pp. 462–466, 09 1952.

67. J. Portilla et al., "Image Denoising Using Gaussian Scale Mixtures in the Wavelet Domain," IEEE Trans. on Image Proc. , Vol. 12, No. 11, 2003, pp. 1338-1351.

68. Jain, Viren, and Sebastian Seung. "Natural image de-noising with convolutional networks." In Advances in Neural Information Proc. Syms, pp. 769-776. 2009.

69. Jamroga, David, Richard J. Friswell, David S. Cook, and Michael K. Patenaude. "Method for storing and accessing digital medical images." U.S. Patent 6,574,742, issued June 3, 2003.

70. Jiang, Jun, Yao Wu, Meiyan Huang, Wei Yang, Wufan Chen, and Qianjin Feng. "3D brain tumor segmentation in multimodal MR images based on learning population-and patient-specific feature sets." Computerized Medical Imaging and Graphics 37, no. 7-8 (2013): 512-521.

71. K. Kamnitsas,W. Bai, E. Ferrante, S. G. McDonagh, M. Sinclair, N. Pawlowski, M. Rajchl, M. C. H. Lee, B. Kainz, D. Rueckert, and B. Glocker, "Ensembles of multiple models and architectures for robust brain tumour segmentation," CoRR, vol. abs/1711.01468, 2017.

72. K. Simonyan and A. Zisserman, "Very deep convolutional networks for large-scale image recognition," in International Conference for Learning Representations, 2015.

73. K. Simonyan and A. Zisserman, "Very deep convolutional networks for large-scale image recognition," in International Conference for Learning Representations, 2015.

74. Kalti, Karim, and Mohamed Ali Mahjoub. "Image segmentation by gaussian mixture models and modified FCM algorithm." Int. Arab J. Inf. Technol. 11, no. 1 (2014): 11-18.

75. Kamdi, Shilpa, and R. K. Krishna. "Image segmentation and region growing algorithm." International Journal of Computer Technology and Electronics Engineering (IJCTEE) 2, no. 1 (2012).

76. Kamnitsas, et al. "Efficient multi-scale 3D CNN with fully connected CRF for accurate brain lesion segmentation." Medical image anal. 36 (2017): 61-78.

77. Kang, Min H., and C. Patrick Reynolds. "Bcl-2 inhibitors: targeting mitochondrial apoptotic pathways in cancer therapy." Clinical cancer research 15, no. 4 (2009): 1126-1132.

78. Kang, Wen-Xiong, Qing-Qiang Yang, and Run-Peng Liang. "The comparative research on image segmentation algorithms." In 2009 First International Workshop on Education Technology and Computer Science, vol. 2, pp. 703-707. IEEE, 2009.

79. Kim, Taehwan, James C. Bezdek, and Richard J. Hathaway. "Optimality tests for fixed points of the fuzzy c-means algorithm." Pattern Recognition 21, no. 6 (1988): 651-663.

80. Kleihues, Paul, and Leslie H. Sobin. "World Health Organization classification of tumors." Cancer 88, no. 12 (2000): 2887-2887ImageNet. http://www.image-net.org

81. Krizhevsky, A., I. Sutskever, and G. E. Hinton. "ImageNet Classification with Deep Convolutional Neural Networks." Advances in Neural Information Processing Systems. Vol 25, 2012.

82. Krizhevsky, Alex, Ilya Sutskever, and Geoffrey E. Hinton. "Imagenet classification with deep convolutional neural networks." In Advances in neural information processing systems, pp. 1097-1105. 2012.

83. Krizhevsky, Alex, Ilya Sutskever, and Geoffrey E. Hinton. "Imagenet classification with deep convolutional neural networks." In Advances in neural information processing systems, pp. 1097-1105. 2012.

84. Lakshmi, A., T. Arivoli, and R. Vinupriyadharshini. "Noise and skull removal of brain magnetic resonance image using curvelet transform and mathematical morphology." In 2014 International Conference on Electronics and Communication Systems (ICECS), pp. 1-4. IEEE, 2014.

85. Lebrun, Marc. "An analysis and implementation of the BM3D image denoising method." Image Processing On Line 2 (2012): 175-213.

86. LeCun, Y., Boser, B., Denker, J.S., Henderson, D., Howard, R.E., Hubbard, W., Jackel, L.D., et al. "Handwritten Digit Recognition with a Back-propagation Network." In Advances of Neural Information Processing Systems, 1990.

87. LeCun, Y., L. Bottou, Y. Bengio, and P. Haffner. "Gradient-based Learning Applied to Document Recognition." Proceedings of the IEEE.Vol 86, pp. 2278–2324, 1998.

88. Lee, Sang Uk, Seok Yoon Chung, and Rae Hong Park. "A comparative performance study of several global thresholding techniques for segmentation." Computer Vision, Graphics, and Image Processing 52, no. 2 (1990): 171-190.

89. Li, Qingneng, et al. "Glioma segmentation using a novel unified algorithm in multimodal MRI images." IEEE Access: 1-1,(2018).

90. Liang, Zhi-Pei, and Paul C. Lauterbur. Principles of magnetic resonance imaging: a signal processing perspective. SPIE Optical Engineering Press, 2000.

91. Linninger, Andreas A., Michalis Xenos, David C. Zhu, MahadevaBharath R. Somayaji, Srinivasa Kondapalli, and Richard D. Penn. "Cerebrospinal fluid flow in the normal and hydrocephalic human brain." IEEE Transactions on Biomedical Engineering 54, no. 2 (2007): 291-302.

92. Litjens, Geert, et al. "A survey on deep learning in medical image analysis." Medical image anal. 42 (2017): 60-88.

93. Liu, Jin, Min Li, Jianxin Wang, Fangxiang Wu, Tianming Liu, and Yi Pan. "A survey of MRI-based brain tumor segmentation methods." Tsinghua Science and Technology 19, no. 6 (2014): 578-595.

94. Liu, Renhao, Lawrence O. Hall, Dmitry B. Goldgof, Mu Zhou, Robert A. Gatenby, and Kaoutar B. Ahmed. "Exploring deep features from brain tumor magnetic resonance images via transfer learning." In 2016 International Joint Conference on Neural Networks (IJCNN), pp. 235-242. IEEE, 2016.

95. Liu, Tianjiao, Shuaining Xie, Jing Yu, Lijuan Niu, and Weidong Sun. "Classification of thyroid nodules in ultrasound images using deep model based transfer learning and hybrid features." In 2017 IEEE International Conference on Acoustics, Speech and Signal Processing (ICASSP), pp. 919-923. IEEE, 2017.

96. Louis, David N., Arie Perry, Guido Reifenberger, Andreas Von Deimling, Dominique Figarella-Branger, Webster K. Cavenee, Hiroko Ohgaki, Otmar D. Wiestler, Paul Kleihues, and David W. Ellison. "The 2016 World Health Organization classification of tumors of the central nervous system: a summary." Acta neuropathologica 131, no. 6 (2016): 803-820.

97. Luisier, Florian, Thierry B, and M.Unser. "Image denoising in mixed Poisson–Gaussian noise." IEEE Trans. on image proc. 20, no. 3 (2011): 696-708.

98. Mao, Xiaojiao, et al., "Image restoration using very deep convolutional encoder-decoder networks with symmetric skip connections." In Advances in neural information proc. syms, pp. 2802-2810. 2016.

99. Marois, Christian, René Doyon, René Racine, and Daniel Nadeau. "Efficient speckle noise attenuation in faint companion imaging." Publications of the Astronomical Society of the Pacific 112, no. 767 (2000): 91.

100. McKinley, Richard, et al. "Ensembles of densely-connected CNNs with label-uncertainty for brain tumor segmentation." In Int. MICCAI Brainlesion Workshop, pp. 456-465. Springer, Cham, 2018.

101. Mehta, Raghav, and Tal Arbel. "3D U-Net for Brain Tumour Segmentation." In Int. MICCAI Brainlesion Workshop, pp. 254-266. Springer, Cham, 2018.

102. Menze, Bjoern H., Andras Jakab, Stefan Bauer, Jayashree Kalpathy-Cramer, Keyvan Farahani, Justin Kirby, Yuliya Burren et al. "The multimodal brain tumor image segmentation benchmark (BRATS)." IEEE transactions on medical imaging 34, no. 10 (2014): 1993-2024.

103. Milletari, Fausto, et al. "V-net: Fully convolutional neural networks for volumetric medical image segmentation." In 2016 4th Int. Conf. on 3D Vision (3DV), pp. 565-571. IEEE, 2016.

104. Mohsen, Heba, El-Sayed A. El-Dahshan, El-Sayed M. El-Horbaty, and Abdel-Badeeh M. Salem. "Classification using deep learning neural networks for brain tumors." Future Computing and Informatics Journal 3, no. 1 (2018): 68-71.

105. Murphy, K. P. Machine Learning: A Probabilistic Perspective. Cambridge, Massachusetts: The MIT Press, 2012.

106. Myronenko, Andriy. "3D MRI brain tumor segmentation using autoencoder regularization." In Int. MICCAI Brainlesion Workshop, pp. 311-320. Springer, Cham, 2018.

107. N. Qian, "On the momentum term in gradient descent learning algorithms.," Neural Networks, vol. 12, no. 1, pp. 145–151, 1999.

108. Nagi, J., F. Ducatelle, G. A. Di Caro, D. Ciresan, U. Meier, A. Giusti, F. Nagi, J. Schmidhuber, L. M. Gambardella. "Max-Pooling Convolutional Neural Networks for Vision-based Hand Gesture Recognition". IEEE International Conference on Signal and Image Processing Applications (ICSIPA2011), 2011.

109. Nair, V. and G. E. Hinton. "Rectified linear units improve restricted boltzmann machines." In Proc. 27th International Conference on Machine Learning, 2010.

110. Nanthagopal, A. Padma, and R. Sukanesh. "Wavelet statistical texture features-based segmentation and classification of brain computed tomography images." IET image processing 7, no. 1 (2013): 25-32.

111. Nasibov, Efendi N., and Gözde Ulutagay. "A new unsupervised approach for fuzzy clustering." Fuzzy Sets and Systems 158, no. 19 (2007): 2118-2133.

112. Ning, Chun-Yu, Shu-fen Liu, and Ming Qu. "Research on removing noise in medical image based on median filter method." In 2009 IEEE International Symposium on IT in Medicine & Education, vol. 1, pp. 384-388. IEEE, 2009.

113. Norman, Berk, Valentina Pedoia, and Sharmila Majumdar. "Use of 2D U-Net convolutional neural networks for automated cartilage and meniscus segmentation of knee MR imaging data to determine relaxometry and morphometry." Radiology 288, no. 1 (2018): 177-185.

114. Omer, Raqib, and Liping Fu. "An automatic image recognition system for winter road surface condition classification." In 13th international IEEE conference on intelligent transportation systems, pp. 1375-1379. IEEE, 2010.

115. Ostrom, Quinn T et al."CBTRUS Statistical Report: Primary Brain and Other Central Nervous System Tumors Diagnosed in the United States in 2012–2016." Neuro-oncology 21, no. Supplement_5 (2019): v1-v100.

116. Othman, M. Fauzi, and M. Ariffanan M. Basri. "Probabilistic neural network for brain tumor classification." In 2011 2nd Int. Conf. on Intelligent Systems, Modelling and Simulation, pp. 136-138. IEEE, 2011.

117. Otsu, Nobuyuki. "A threshold selection method from gray-level histograms." IEEE transactions on systems, man, and cybernetics 9, no. 1 (1979): 62-66.

118. Pan, Sinno Jialin, and Qiang Yang. "A survey on transfer learning." IEEE Transactions on knowledge and data engineering 22, no. 10 (2010): 1345-1359.

119. Patel, Jay, and Kaushal Doshi. "A study of segmentation methods for detection of tumor in brain MRI." Advance in Electronic and Electric Engineering 4, no. 3 (2014): 279-284.

120. Pereira, Sérgio, et al. "Brain tumor segmentation using convolutional neural networks in MRI images." IEEE trans. medical imaging 35, no. 5 (2016): 1240-1251.

121. Pham, Dzung L., Chenyang Xu, and Jerry L. Prince. "Current methods in medical image segmentation." Annual review of biomedical engineering 2, no. 1 (2000): 315-337.

122. Ponomarenko, Nikolay, Vladimir Lukin, Mikhail Zriakhov, Karen Egiazarian, and Jaakko Astola. "Lossy compression of images with additive noise." In International Conference on Advanced Concepts for Intelligent Vision Systems, pp. 381-386. Springer, Berlin, Heidelberg, 2005.

123. Prajapati, Shreyansh A., R. Nagaraj, and Suman Mitra. "Classification of dental diseases using CNN and transfer learning." In 2017 5th International Symposium on Computational and Business Intelligence (ISCBI), pp. 70-74. IEEE, 2017.

124. Prastawa, Marcel, Elizabeth Bullitt, Sean Ho, and Guido Gerig. "A brain tumor segmentation framework based on outlier detection." Medical image analysis 8, no. 3 (2004): 275-283.

125. Qassim, Hussam, Abhishek Verma, and David Feinzimer. "Compressed residual-VGG16 CNN model for big data places image recognition." In 2018 IEEE 8th Annual Computing and Communication Workshop and Conference (CCWC), pp. 169-175. IEEE, 2018.

126. R. S. Sutton, "Two problems with backpropagation and other steepest-descent learning procedures for networks," in Proceedings of the Eighth Annual Conference of the Cognitive Science Society, Hillsdale, NJ: Erlbaum, 1986.

127. Ronneberger, et al. "U-net: Convolutional networks for biomedical image segmentation." In Int. Conf. on Medical image computing and computer-assisted intervention, pp. 234-241. Springer, Cham, 2015.

128. Roslan, Rosniza, Nursuriati Jamil, and Rozi Mahmud. "Skull stripping magnetic resonance images brain images: region growing versus mathematical morphology." International Journal of Computer Information Systems and Industrial Management Applications 3 (2011): 150-158.

129. Russakovsky, O., Deng, J., Su, H., et al. "ImageNet Large Scale Visual Recognition Challenge." International Journal of Computer Vision (IJCV). Vol 115, Issue 3, 2015, pp. 211–252

130. Russakovsky, Olga, Jia Deng, Hao Su, Jonathan Krause, Sanjeev Satheesh, Sean Ma, Zhiheng Huang et al. "Imagenet large scale visual recognition challenge." International journal of computer vision 115, no. 3 (2015): 211-252.

131. S. Gu, et al, "Weighted nuclear norm minimization with application to image de-noising," in IEEE Conf. on Computer Vision and Pattern Recognition, pp. 2862–2869, 2014.

132. Sachdeva, Jainy, Vinod Kumar, Indra Gupta, Niranjan Khandelwal, and Chirag Kamal Ahuja. "Multiclass brain tumor classification using GA-SVM." In 2011 Developments in E-systems Engineering, pp. 182-187. IEEE, 2011.

133. Salmon, Joseph, Zachary Harmany, Charles-Alban Deledalle, and Rebecca Willett. "Poisson noise reduction with non-local PCA." Journal of mathematical imaging and vision 48, no. 2 (2014): 279-294.

134. Sampat, Mehul P., Mia K. Markey, and Alan C. Bovik. "Computer-aided detection and diagnosis in mammography." Handbook of image and video processing 2, no. 1 (2005): 1195-1217.

135. Sebastian, V., A. Unnikrishnan, and K. Balakrishnan. "Gray level co-occurrence matrices: generalisation and some new features." arXiv preprint arXiv:1205.4831 (2012).

136. Seetha, J., and S. Selvakumar Raja. "Brain tumor classification using convolutional neural networks." Biomedical & Pharmacology Journal 11, no. 3 (2018): 1457.

137. Sezgin, Mehmet, and Bülent Sankur. "Survey over image thresholding techniques and quantitative performance evaluation." Journal of Electronic imaging 13, no. 1 (2004): 146-166.

138. Shafarenko, Leila, Maria Petrou, and Josef Kittler. "Automatic watershed segmentation of randomly textured color images." IEEE transactions on Image Processing 6, no. 11 (1997): 1530-1544.

139. Sharma, Minakshi, and Sourabh Mukharjee. "Brain tumor segmentation using hybrid genetic algorithm and artificial neural network fuzzy inference system (anfis)." International Journal of Fuzzy Logic Systems 2, no. 4 (2012): 31-42.

140. Shin, Hoo-Chang et al., "Deep convolutional neural networks for computer-aided detection: CNN architectures, dataset characteristics and transfer learning." IEEE transactions on medical imaging 35, no. 5 (2016): 1285-1298.

141. Silbergeld, Daniel L., and Michael R. Chicoine. "Isolation and characterization of human malignant glioma cells from histologically normal brain." Journal of neurosurgery 86, no. 3 (1997): 525-531.

142. Srimani, P. K., and Shanthi Mahesh. "A Comparative study of different segmentation techniques for brain tumour detection." International journal of emerging technologies in computational and applied sciences 2, no. 4 (2013): 192-197.

143. Srivastava, N., G. Hinton, A. Krizhevsky, I. Sutskever, R. Salakhutdinov. "Dropout: A Simple Way to Prevent Neural Networks from Overfitting." Journal of Machine Learning Research. Vol. 15, pp. 1929-1958, 2014.

144. Stawiaski, Jean. "A Pretrained DenseNet Encoder for Brain Tumor Segmentation." In Int. MICCAI Brainlesion Workshop, pp. 105-115. Springer, Cham, 2018.

145. Sudre, Carole H., M. Jorge Cardoso, Willem H. Bouvy, Geert Jan Biessels, Josephine Barnes, and Sebastien Ourselin. "Bayesian model selection for pathological neuroimaging data applied to white matter lesion segmentation." IEEE transactions on medical imaging 34, no. 10 (2015): 2079-2102.

146. Suganthi, P. Deepaland M., and P. Deepa. "Performance evaluation of various denoising filters for medical image." International journal of computer science and information Technologies 5, no. 3 (2014): 4205-4209.

147. Sun, Xiaolong, Juyoung P., K. Kang, and Junbeom Hur. "Novel hybrid CNN-SVM model for recognition of functional magnetic resonance images." In 2017 IEEE Int. Conf. on Systems, Man, and Cybernetics (SMC), pp. 1001-1006. IEEE, 2017.

148. Surawicz, Tanya S., Bridget J. McCarthy, Varant Kupelian, Patti J. Jukich, Janet M. Bruner, and Faith G. Davis. "Descriptive epidemiology of primary brain and CNS tumors: results from the Central Brain Tumor Registry of the United States, 1990-1994." Neuro-oncology 1, no. 1 (1999): 14-25.

149. Suter, Yannick, Alain Jungo, Michael Rebsamen, Urspeter Knecht, Evelyn Herrmann, Roland Wiest, and Mauricio Reyes. "Deep Learning versus Classical Regression for Brain Tumor Patient Survival Prediction." In International MICCAI Brainlesion Workshop, pp. 429-440. Springer, Cham, 2018.

150. Swati, Zar Nawab Khan, Qinghua Zhao, Muhammad Kabir, Farman Ali, Zakir Ali, Saeed Ahmed, and Jianfeng Lu. "Brain tumor classification for MR images using transfer learning and fine-tuning." Computerized Medical Imaging and Graphics 75 (2019): 34-46.

151. Szilagyi, Laszlo, Zoltan Benyo, Sandor M. Szilagyi, and H. S. Adam. "MR brain image segmentation using an enhanced fuzzy c-means algorithm." In Proceedings of the 25th Annual International Conference of the IEEE Engineering in Medicine and Biology Society (IEEE Cat. No. 03CH37439), vol. 1, pp. 724-726. IEEE, 2003.

152. Szkulmowski, Maciej, Iwona Gorczynska, Daniel Szlag, Marcin Sylwestrzak, Andrzej Kowalczyk, and Maciej Wojtkowski. "Efficient reduction of speckle noise in Optical Coherence Tomography." Optics express 20, no. 2 (2012): 1337-1359.

153. Talo, Muhammed, Ulas Baran Baloglu, Özal Yıldırım, and U. Rajendra Acharya. "Application of deep transfer learning for automated brain abnormality classification using MR images." Cognitive Systems Research 54 (2019): 176-188.

154. Tang, Jinshan, Shengwen Guo, Qingling Sun, Youping Deng, and Dongfeng Zhou. "Speckle reducing bilateral filter for cattle follicle segmentation." BMC genomics 11, no. 2 (2010): S9.

155. Tilton, James C., Yuliya Tarabalka, Paul M. Montesano, and Emanuel Gofman. "Best merge region-growing segmentation with integrated nonadjacent region object aggregation." IEEE Transactions on Geoscience and Remote Sensing 50, no. 11 (2012): 4454-4467.

156. Torbati, Nima, Ahmad Ayatollahi, and Ali Kermani. "An efficient neural network based method for medical image segmentation." Computers in biology and medicine 44 (2014): 76-87.

157. Torrey, Lisa, and Jude Shavlik. "Transfer learning." In Handbook of Research on Machine Learning Applications and Trends: Algorithms, Methods, and Techniques, pp. 242-264. IGI Global, 2010.

158. Travis, William D., Elisabeth Brambilla, Andrew G. Nicholson, Yasushi Yatabe, John HM Austin, Mary Beth Beasley, Lucian R. Chirieac et al. "The 2015 World Health Organization classification of lung tumors: impact of genetic, clinical and radiologic advances since the 2004 classification." Journal of thoracic oncology 10, no. 9 (2015): 1243-1260.

159. Unterberg, A. W., J. Stover, B. Kress, and K. L. Kiening. "Edema and brain trauma." Neuroscience 129, no. 4 (2004): 1019-1027.

160. Van De Ville, Dimitri, Mike Nachtegael, Dietrich Van der Weken, Etienne E. Kerre, Wilfried Philips, and Ignace Lemahieu. "Noise reduction by fuzzy image filtering." IEEE transactions on fuzzy systems 11, no. 4 (2003): 429-436.

161. W. Dong, L. Zhang, G. Shi, and X. Li, "Nonlocally centralized sparse representation for image restoration," IEEE Transactions on Image Processing, vol. 22, no. 4, pp. 1620–1630, 2013.

162. W. McCulloch and W. Pitts, "A logical calculus of ideas immanent in nervous activity," Bulletin of Mathematical Biophysics, vol. 5, pp. 115–133, 1943.

163. Wagstaff, Kiri, Claire Cardie, Seth Rogers, and Stefan Schrödl. "Constrained k-means clustering with background knowledge." In Icml, vol. 1, pp. 577-584. 2001.

164. Wang, Qi, Xiang He, and Xuelong Li. "Locality and structure regularized low rank representation for hyperspectral image classification." IEEE Transactions on Geoscience and Remote Sensing 57, no. 2 (2018): 911-923.

165. Wang, Qing et al. "Heterogeneity Diffusion Imaging of gliomas: Initial experience and validation." PloS one 14, no. 11 (2019).

166. Weidle, Ulrich H., JENS NIEWÖHNER, and Georg Tiefenthaler. "The blood–brain barrier challenge for the treatment of brain cancer, secondary brain metastases, and neurological diseases." Cancer Genomics-Proteomics 12, no. 4 (2015): 167-177.

167. Xiao-Ping Zhang, "Thresholding Neural Network for Adaptive Noise Reduction." IEEE Transactions on Neural Networks, Vol. 12, No. 3, May 2001.

168. Xu, Yan, Zhipeng Jia, Yuqing Ai, Fang Zhang, Maode Lai, I. Eric, and Chao Chang. "Deep convolutional activation features for large scale brain tumor histopathology image classification and segmentation." In 2015 IEEE international conference on acoustics, speech and signal processing (ICASSP), pp. 947-951. IEEE, 2015.

169. Y. LeCun, L. Bottou, Y. Bengio, and P. Haffner, "Gradient-based learning applied to document recognition," Proceedings of the IEEE, vol. 86, no. 11, pp. 2278–2324, 1998.

170. Yang, Tiejun, Jikun Song, and Lei Li. "A deep learning model integrating SK-TPCNN and random forests for brain tumor segmentation in MRI." Biocybernetics and Biomedical Engg. (2019).

171. Zacharaki, Evangelia I., Sumei Wang, Sanjeev Chawla, Dong Soo Yoo, Ronald Wolf, Elias R. Melhem, and Christos Davatzikos. "Classification of brain tumor type and grade using MRI texture and shape in a machine learning scheme." Magnetic Resonance in Medicine: An Official Journal of the International Society for Magnetic Resonance in Medicine 62, no. 6 (2009): 1609-1618.

172. Zhang, Jun, and Jinglu Hu. "Image segmentation based on 2D Otsu method with histogram analysis." In 2008 International Conference on Computer Science and Software Engineering, vol. 6, pp. 105-108. IEEE, 2008.

173. Zhang, Kai et al., "Beyond a gaussian denoiser: Residual learning of deep cnn for image denoising." IEEE Trans. on Image Proc. 26, no. 7 (2017): 3142-3155.

174. Zhang, Kai, Wangmeng Zuo, and Lei Zhang. "FFDNet: Toward a fast and flexible solution for CNN-based image denoising." IEEE Transactions on Image Processing 27, no. 9 (2018): 4608-4622.

175. Zhang, Kai, Wangmeng Zuo, Yunjin Chen, Deyu Meng, and Lei Zhang. "Beyond a gaussian denoiser: Residual learning of deep cnn for image denoising." IEEE Transactions on Image Processing 26, no. 7 (2017): 3142-3155.

176. Zhang, Ming, and Bahadir K. Gunturk. "Multiresolution bilateral filtering for image de-noising." IEEE Trans. on image proc. 17, no. 12 (2008): 2324-2333.

177. Zhang, Yu-Dong, et al., "Magnetic resonance brain image classification based on weighted-type fractional Fourier transform and nonparallel support vector machine." Inter Jour. of Imaging Systems and Technology 25, no. 4 (2015): 317-327.

178. Zhang, Yu-Dong, Lenan Wu, and Shuihua Wang. "Magnetic resonance brain image classification by an improved artificial bee colony algorithm." Progress In Electromagnetics Research 116 (2011): 65-79.

179. Zhu, Xiaojin, and Andrew B. Goldberg. "Introduction to semi-supervised learning." Synthesis lectures on artificial intelligence and machine learning 3, no. 1 (2009): 1-130.

180. Ziou, Djemel, and Salvatore Tabbone. "Edge detection techniques-an overview." Pattern Recognition and Image Analysis C/C of Raspoznavaniye Obrazov I Analiz Izobrazhenii 8 (1998): 537-559.

181. Zoran, Daniel, and Yair Weiss. "From learning models of natural image patches to whole image restoration." In 2011 International Conference on Computer Vision, pp. 479-486. IEEE, 2011.

Chapter 6

Conclusions and Future Scope of the Work

Tumors can be benign (Noncancerous) or malignant (Cancerous) which have different features and can be identified through brain tumor MR imaging. Different standards for grading of tumors are given by World Health Organization (WHO) and a grade indicates the severity of the tumor. Doctors may identify the type of tumor based on the observations in the brain tumor images and accordingly plan for effective treatment. The BraTS 2018 database is used for training and evaluation of model performance. In this database, the structural information (subregions) and their labels of brain tumor MR images for segmentation task are discussed. (Ch.2).

The performance of PSNR for Gaussian noise corrupted image is improved to 14.24 % in the proposed DeepCNN model for a noise level of 5 and an improvement of 7.66 % is achieved with speckle noise addition. For a Gaussian noise with known noise level of 15, the proposed DeepCNN model shows an improvement of PSNR in dB of 8.39 %. The proposed DeepCNN model appears to be better for reducing noise when image gets corrupted by either speckle or Gaussian noise with known or unknown noise levels. In addition, the proposed DeepCNN preserves the structural information of the image by observing the SSIM values from the results. (Ch.3).

The proposed Transfer Learning model considered for classification of brain tumor MR images is much faster and easier when compared to hybrid models. The proposed TL with ADAM optimizer has obtained an accuracy of 97.91 % with an error rate of 2.08 %. Proposed TL with SGDM optimizer and proposed hybrid CNN-KNN model achieved same accuracy of 96.25 % with an error rate of 3.75 %. An improvement of 1.71 % in accuracy is obtained for proposed TL with ADAM optimizer when compared to the proposed TL with SGDM optimizer and hybrid models respectively. An improvement of error rate of 80.29 % is achieved considering proposed TL with ADAM optimizer when compared to the proposed TL with SGDM optimizer and hybrid models respectively. Hence, the proposed TL model can be used for early detection and classification of brain tumor which will increase the chances of treatment and curing the patients effectively. (Ch.4)

Segmentation of brain tumor glioma subregions is performed using two proposed DL models. With the 23 layer deep learning model, an average accuracy of 98.20 %, 98.81 %, 99.74 % and average error rate of 1.79 %, 1.19 %, and 0.26 % are achieved for whole tumor extraction using K-means, Fuzzy C-means and DL model respectively. The extracted whole tumor is further used with an 18 layer DL model and T1c image to obtain the subregions ET and TC. The performance of the proposed models are evaluated on parameters like accuracy, error rate, sensitivity, specificity, F1-measure, dice similarity coefficient, and Jaccard similarity coefficient. An average dice coefficients of 0.96702, 0.9281, 0.9152, and Jaccard coefficients of 0.9374, 0.8835, 0.8471 and an accuracy of 99.82 %, 99.88 %, and 99.73 %, are attained for ET, TC, and WT respectively. (Ch.5).

Future Scope

As a result of the investigations carried out in this thesis, the following aspects will provide the scope for extending this work to the next level. To detect various types of tumor in all the parts of human body like liver, breast, lungs, etc. and also the work can be extended to find the patient survival rate; the work can also be useful for disease detection in plant leaves and cropping, applying data augmentation transformation to model enlarges the database in order to avoid over-fitting problems advanced pretrained CNN model can be used for faster implementation and better accuracy can be achieved through further tuning of hyper parameters and also develop new network architectures with custom loss function to improve the performance.

CPSIA information can be obtained
at www.ICGtesting.com
Printed in the USA
BVHW052359270623
666449BV00016B/750